Here's what others are saying about

Stress Express!
by Snowden McFall

"As a busy mom of four and home-based business owner, speaker, author, PTA President, church member...(you get the idea), I was excited to get my hands on this book. Full of great examples and actionable ideas, I can immediately implement several of these practical suggestions for decreasing my stress level! (The chapter on optimism alone is worth the price of the book!)"

Carrie Wilkerson,
Author of *The Barefoot Executive*

"Wise advice from a very wise teacher regarding one of the most vital and important aspects of our life. Listen to Snowden and live a life much less stressful… and much more joyful."

Bob Burg
Co-Author of *The Go-Giver and Go-Givers Sell More*
Author of *Endless Referrals*

"I love this book. Snowden shares valuable insights and current data on ways to relieve stress in a fascinating and delightful manner. Her stories and photos underscore the latest research on stress and what each of us can do to be healthier and happier. You definitely want this book; you'll refer to it over and over again."

Pegine Echevarria, MSW
Motivational Speakers Hall of Fame Inductee and Author

"I just loved Stress Express! Terrific ideas for reducing and managing stress! As a business owner, there's never enough time in the day to handle all the challenges of daily life. Snowden offers practical tips in a concise style, with actionable items that are manageable yet effective. I especially enjoyed Stress Reliever #14 related to Optimism. I now keep a copy on my nightstand as a handy reference."

Deborah Eveson,
Eveson Allstate Insurance Agency

Stress Express!

15 Instant Stress Relievers

SNOWDEN McFALL

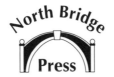

Stress Express!

15 Instant Stress Relievers

Snowden McFall

Copyright ©2010, 2014 by Snowden McFall
Published by North Bridge Press, Jacksonville, FL

Library of Congress Cataloging in Publication

Preassigned LCCN: 2010928743
ISBN 9781892372024

Other data is available from the Library of Congress

Manufactured in the United States of America

Acknowledgements

This book has been a long process over several years, and there are so many people who have encouraged me along the way. My editorial team has been fantastic, often working with very tight deadlines. Editor Patti D'Addieco has been wonderful. Alice Howard, Joe Montano, Spencer Whiting, many thanks for eagle eye proofing and feedback. Kudos to cover designer Kawise Mack, with fine tuning by Tom Agriesti with last minute changes.

Tanya Guydos of Florida Bank, thank you for your kind generosity and support of hosting my booksigning party, and 30th anniversary party. Dana Stallings, thanks for the chocolate *Stress Express!* basket. Dear friends Barbara Moulding, Diane Longo, Camille Gregg, Kim Lambert, Elizabeth Paulson, Teri Tompkins, Tammy Wainright, Denise Thomas, Skip and Judy Jackson, Felina Martin, Nancy and Dom Grasso, Ed and Denise Conmey, Jeri Silver Miller, and Stawn Barber, I love and appreciate you. Your encouragement and ideas were so valuable.

The many women's groups I belong to always lift my spirits. Professional Women's Council, Women Business Owners, Jacksonville Women's Network and more, thank you for the learning and friendships.

Carrie Wilkerson, Bob Burg, Pegine Echevarria, Joe Montano, Richard Hadden, Chris Morris, Deb Eveson, and Jeannie Fredrick, thank you for your kind endorsements.

I am so blessed to have a wonderful, loving husband. Spencer, you cheered me at every turn, even when it seemed I had to experience the stress I wrote about. You are my best friend and I love you.

John Roger and John Morton, you have been amazing teachers and gifts to me. I can never begin to thank you for the love, the light and the constant learning I receive from you. I love you.

And finally, I wish to thank God, who made it very clear to me that it was time to write this book. Thank you for your constant, guiding presence in my life and all the learnings and lessons, blessings and miracles, grace and gifts.

Contents

Introduction
Why a Stress Book? Why Now?

The answer is that **stress is epidemic**, and it is literally killing people all over the world. From the Japanese term "karoshi," which means death by overwork, to the startling statistics on the impact of stress worldwide, it is clear that we must tackle our stress in order to live more fulfilling and healthy lives.

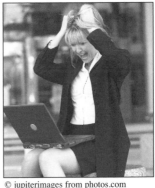

© jupiterimages from photos.com

Personally and corporately, **stress is one of the most expensive factors in the workplace today,** worldwide. The American Psychological Association says stress costs industry $300 billion a year in absences, medical costs, lost productivity, turnover etc. Medical costs in the US are skyrocketing, expected to reach $4.8 trillion in 2021.[1a] Stress-related claims cost US companies 10% of their annual earnings. A typical employee with stress, back pain and depression is out of work nine weeks a year and can cost more than $5900 per employee in lost productivity.[1] The numbers around the world are equally staggering.

Work is often the culprit, although financial woes are a strong issue for many. Think about your life and those of your friends and neighbors. How many are working long, hard hours for less? Are any unemployed or sick? How about you? How stressful is your career? Do you look forward to your job or do you dread going to work? If you're stressed, you're not alone.

One third of Americans say they are living with extreme stress.[2] A study done by Career Builder.com says that 78% of all American workers feel burned out. The American Psychological Asssociation's 2013 study found that 1/3 of Americans experience chronic work stress.

The Impact of Stress at Work

2/3 of Americans say work has a significant impact on their stress levels. With cutbacks, layoffs, economic pressures and reduced spending, most workplaces are just not as much fun as they used to be. Most employees dread going to work. Think about your life. Do you love your job? Do you look forward to going to work? Or are you tired, irritable, frustrated and ready to leave at 3:00?

60% of work absences are due to psychological issues such as fear of layoff, stress and burnout. The Bureau of National Affairs states that 40% of all job turnover is due to stress. [3]

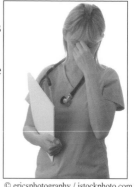

Stressed employees mean poorer performance in the office. That creates a vicious cycle of declining productivity and lower sales. Then there is more pressure and people are even more stressed and unhappy. Gallup says that 80% of all Americans feel work stress and 50% need help managing it. The Gallup Management Journal found that nearly **20 million workers are actively "disengaged."** Another 70

© ericsphotography / istockphoto.com

million are not engaged; they are simply present. (Disengaged employees are not enthusiastic, motivated hard workers; they simply don't care anymore.) Disengaged employees miss more days of work annually (86.5 million) than other workers. More importantly, disengaged employees are not productive, effective and creative in the workplace.

What about you? Are you fired up about your job and your workplace? Do

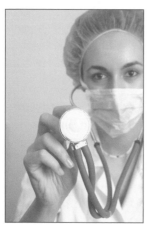

you look forward to each day? When you're exhausted and unhappy with your job, how do you feel when you get a new project? Excited, challenged, delighted? Most people these days just groan or scream inwardly, and wonder how they will ever get through the day, much less through a new project.

Stress and Your Health

Stress takes a tremendous toll on your body. According to the American Psychological Association:

• nearly 80% of all doctor visits are stress-related

© Olaru Radian-alexandru /

• 43% of all adults have ill health because of stress.

Stress is linked to the six major causes of death: heart disease, cancer, lung disease, accidents, cirrhosis, and suicide.[4] Financial concerns over health are a major source of stress for many families around the world.

Knowledge is power. If you know how stress can hurt your body, you are much more likely to take care of yourself and monitor your stress levels. Stress impacts health on so many levels. Heart disease is the #1 cause of death in women over 40 and it is a leading cause of death in men. It takes a life every 34 seconds and affects over 80 million people. It kills more people in the US than anything else, and is aggravated by stress. Here's the good news: **you can be proactive about preventing heart disease by using stress relief strategies, eating better,**

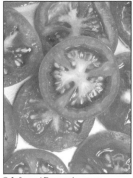
© Infocus / Dreamstime.com

and exercising regularly. If your family has a history of heart disease, you can learn the key indicators and monitor your heart with your physician. You can eat heart-healthy foods, reduce your stress and stay well.

The second biggest killer of both men and women is cancer, which is worsened (and some say caused) by stress. Dr. Eric Yang from the James Cancer Hospital and Solove Research Institute says "*studies have shown that psychological stress affects the immune system, and in that way, that's the mechanism by which cancers are able to progress.*" Here's the good news: recent studies by Dr. Yang have demonstrated that reducing stress can prevent cancer's recurrence. Using betablockers to suppress stress has kept tumors from growing and may prevent many cancers. That means you can help prevent cancer from recurring by reducing stress.[5] Consult your physician about this new research.

The Best News of All: We CAN Relieve, Manage and Prevent Stress

All over the world, **studies on stress management and wellness programs show they pay huge dividends in health, productivity, and cost-savings**. Companies with work-life policies and stress management programs see a dramatic decrease in employee turnover.[6] Here are other notable findings:

• If 100 people eliminate three unhealthy stress and health-related behaviors, an employer can see an annual savings of $448,000.[7] What unhealthy behavior could you eliminate? Poor eating? Not exercising? Getting too little sleep?

• Stress management and employee wellness programs can see a return of $3-6 for every dollar invested over a 2-5 year period. Savings show in decreased absenteeism, workers' comp claims, medical costs, and short-term disability.[8]

• A Duke University study shows that stress management reduced the chance that heart patients will have another cardiac event. And costs related to those patients were **cut in half** when they used stress management.[9] So if you have heart problems, stress management can make a huge difference to you.

- IBM found that on average, healthcare costs for those who exercise 1-2 times a week are $350 less a year than those who don't exercise.[10]

- Coors Brewing Company found that absenteeism dropped 18% with its wellness programs.[11]

- Johnson and Johnson's wellness and stress management program reduced cholesterol levels, blood pressure and cut smoking with a dollar savings of **$8.8 million annually**.[12]

- An analysis of the records of 22,838 subjects enrolled in Citibank's Health Management Program indicates a corporate wellness ROI of between $4.56 and $4.73 per dollar spent on the program.[13] If you own a small business, think of what a stress management program could save *your* company.

All of the people who work at these companies and participate in their stress management programs reap the benefits. What about you? Do you have a gym at work that you could use more often? Stress management and wellness programs that cost you nothing? Yoga and exercise classes that are free? Take advantage of every chance you get to become healthier.

So What Does it Take to Reduce Your Stress?

The answer is not that much. **About 15 - 30 minutes a day of using various stress relief techniques can make a huge difference.** Whether you are deep breathing, exercising, reading, getting more sleep, laughing, meditating or spending time with friends, **you have the power to change** your habits, reduce your stress and potentially save your own life.

That's why I wrote this book. I have been studying stress for over 15 years. In many respects, it is the flip side of being *Fired Up!* (my first book) because it leads to burnout. I have been researching stress studies and specific stress management techniques, and their results at length. As I travel around the U.S., speaking to corporations, associations, entrepreneurs, and professional women, it has become clear that everyone wants something quick, easy and effective that they can apply to their lives immediately. That's the foundation of *Stress Express! 15 Instant Stress Relievers*. My goal is to give you practical, effective and quick tips: tools you can use right now in this moment to reduce stress.

So let's get started. Flip through the book to any chapter that appeals to you. Read the stories designated by the little clock icon and see if you can relate. Study the various practical tips provided and try one out. You may be surprised by some, but everything here is research-backed (as you can see from the extensive footnotes.) Check it out for yourself and use what works best for you. You deserve a life where you feel joyful, radiantly healthy and vibrantly alive. You deserve to be *Fired Up!* rather than burnt-out! It's all your choice.

Preface

Someone asked me if I felt I had to create more stress in my life in order to write this book, and on some level, I must have, because the year in which I first wrote this was very stressful. There were times I was truly close to burnout, so I can honestly say, I can empathize with that feeling.

One of the biggest stressors came from the loss of a courageous and lovely woman, Gretchen Whiting, my sister-in-law. After several years of bravely battling melanoma, she died at age 41, leaving behind her husband Ren and young son Jack. For years, Gretchen had been a major fundraiser for the Fred Hutchinson Cancer Center in Seattle. After her death, Ren and Gretchen's entire families and friends (including me and my husband) gathered to walk in the Hutch's Shore Run/Walk, raising over $47,000. Gretchen's photo throughout the walk reminded us of her impact.

Sadly, Gretchen was just one of several people in my life with cancer. I still have two very dear friends who are cheerfully and confidently battling cancer every day, defying dire predictions of early demises. Your constant courage, tenacity and love of life humble me.

Like many of you, my businesses were negatively impacted by the economy and so was my husband's. That made financial stress a factor in our lives on a greater level than before.

Two of my great loves are my wonderful cats, Trinity and Gabriel. Unfortunately, Trinity swallowed some strapping tape and ended up with a bacterial infection in her gall bladder, which has resulted in all sorts of health issues. It's so sad when animals or small children are sick, because it's hard to know where their pain is and how best to comfort them. My kitties are such a huge source of stress relief for me that I want to shower them with all the love I can.

And just a few years ago, I lost four people in the space of three months. Cinderella, the wonderful woman who raised me, died along with my first cousin, a young dear friend and my father. Death and dying is stressful, and grief can be difficult to overcome. The tools in this book helped me.

I have tried personally almost everything in this book to reduce my stress and improve my health and well-being. It is my heart's wish that you apply these same techniques and tips and live a less stressful, more joyful life.

Are You on the Edge of Burn-Out?
A Quick Test

Check any that apply to you right now:

❑ You come home regularly dead-tired with little or no energy.

❑ You stay awake at night thinking about all the things you have to do.

❑ The concept of vacation is inconceivable to you- you have way too much to do to go away.

❑ You don't have time to exercise regularly or participate in your favorite hobbies.

❑ You don't have time for massages, haircuts, or personal care like doctor's and dentist's appointments.

❑ You snap at your loved ones and co-workers fairly often.

❑ You have very little patience with others and expect them to work as hard as you do.

❑ You are very critical, especially of yourself.

❑ You feel your life is out of control.

❑ You eat on the fly, often junk or fast food.

❑ You don't like change and wish things were how they once were.

❑ You feel unappreciated, unloved and undervalued.

If you checked 5 or more, you could be heading towards burnout.
Look on the next page for some instant stress relievers to help get balance back into your life.

Instant Stress Reliever # 1 Relax Your Jaw
Tooth Grinding and Jaw Clenching are
a Real Headache - Literally!

"Holding on to anger, resentment and hurt only gives you tense muscles, a headache and a sore jaw from clenching your teeth. Forgiveness gives you back the laughter and the lightness in your life."
Joan Lunden

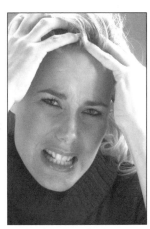

© pidjoe / istockphoto.com

Right now, check your neck and shoulders. Any tension there? How about if you put your fingers right behind the bottom of your ears? Is it at all sore? Now put your fingers at the spot about two inches below your temples where your upper and lower jaw meet. Is it tight? We all express our stress in creative ways and for far too many of us, it can show up in the form of jaw pain, a result of clenching your jaw or grinding your teeth at night.

Believe it or not, a clenched jaw exerts up to **600 pounds** of pressure, which can damage your teeth, gums and fillings.[1] Dentists all over the world are reporting that more and more people are grinding their teeth than ever before, probably because of the economy. Some dentists report the incidents have doubled.

Why is this a problem? Teeth grinding itself, known as "bruxism," can wear down your teeth, **crack them or reduce cusps to flat stumps**. Repair is very costly, often in the thousands of dollars. Over time, continuous jaw clenching and teeth grinding can lead to headaches, neck and shoulder pain, and TMJ, (temporomandibular joint & muscle disorder.) TMJ is characterized by clicking or popping of the jaw resulting from a misaligned bite. Severe cases of TMJ can cause the sound of bells ringing in your ears or hearing loss.[2] Some people end up with migraine headaches, sinus infections and tooth abscesses. Another medical side effect of severe clenching and tooth grinding is vertigo, a strong loss of balance that makes it hard to stand. Dr. Curtis Barmby says, "It's the Clint Eastwood muscle" referencing the well-known American actor. "When people are stressed,...the shoulders go up, the teeth come together and the head comes forward." [3] How about you? Have you ever had a very sore jaw or radiating pain from your jaw down your neck, or felt like your teeth were raw from grinding? It's much more common than you would think.

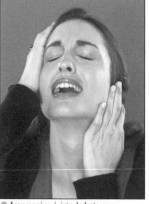

© Juanmonino / istockphoto.com

🕐 *Years ago, I discovered that much of my neck and shoulder pain had an unusual source: bruxism. My massage therapist told me I was clenching my jaw and grinding my teeth at night, and that tension went straight from my jaw to my neck and shoulders. The pain was surprisingly intense. This constant night clenching had created TMJ, a condition I still work with, through massage and natural remedies. I tried a night guard, which works well for many people. I now take the homeopathic remedy Belladonna before bed and it helps me a great deal. (Consult your physician first.) I can always tell when I have forgotten to take it because my mouth and jaw ache in the morning. A short while ago, I woke up with a throbbing headache and very sore chin from having ground my teeth so much that I aggravated my gums. This made my chin swell and created pain that persisted for nearly a week! OWW!*

When Does Bruxism Happen?

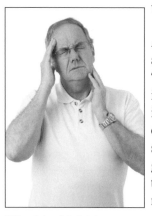

© Steve Luker / istockphoto.com

According to Dr. Lee Weinstein, "bruxism almost always occurs in the shallow dream states of sleep." "If you are bruxing when you would normally go into REM, the action of bruxing can delay your ability to get into REM, thus compromising the amount of REM sleep you get."[4] REM sleep is the deep sleep that rejuvenates us, so if clenching and grinding prevent us from getting REM sleep, there are serious health consequences, including mental illness.

Solutions to Bruxism or Teeth Grinding

So what can you do about it? First, check with your dentist, cranio-sacral specialist, and massage therapist to see if you have a problem with teeth grinding or TMJ. Your dentist will be able to see a wearing down on your teeth, and check if there is a jaw misalignment. You may need to repair cracked teeth. Your dentist will probably recommend getting a custom fit night guard. You can also buy one yourself at a drugstore and examine it after a few nights to see if you are grinding.

🕐 *A night guard made a big difference for Susan Wittstock, of Berkeley, CA. Having suffered from bruxism for 30 years, she had a chipped front tooth and crack in one of her molars. She was fitted for a guard in 2007 and now is much improved. "Before using it, it would feel like someone had taken a two-by four and whacked me," she said. This led to terrible headaches that lasted for days.*[5]

According to studies at Tufts University, magnesium citrate can help, as well as anti-inflammatories and muscle relaxants.[6] And if it is really bad, a dentist, chiropractor, or cranial-sacral therapist can usually activate trigger points to relieve the strain. Always consult your medical professional.

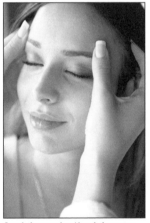
© webphotographer / istockphoto.com

Instant Stress Reliever #1 The Tongue Behind Your Teeth Trick

I've been using it myself this year with great success. Put your fingers behind and just below your ears. If you have tension there, try this. Put your tongue on the roof of your mouth right behind your front teeth. This automatically forces you to relax your jaw and release tension. Do it several times a day and feel how your neck tension subsides.

Instant Stress Reliever #2 Massage the Face

Massage definitely makes a big difference. Massaging the scalp (strange as it seems) helps relieve jaw tension. Grab a fistful of hair on top of your head, gently. If it hurts a great deal, you have jaw tension. Slowly massage and relax your scalp. (Better yet, get someone else to do it for you!)

🕐 *Massage your facial muscles, especially where your jaw opens and closes back towards your ear and under your cheekbones. My husband is wonderful at gentle deep massage on my jaw, stroking and moving out towards my nose, because sometimes the tension lodges in different places. Try this yourself and see how much better you feel.*

Instant Stress Reliever # 3 Hot / Cold Compresses

Alternate treating your pain with ice and heat. Put an icepack on your jaw and cheekbones for 10-15 seconds. Then warm a wet washcloth for 60 seconds. (Be careful not to make it too hot!) Hold it next to your cheek in front of your earlobes to relax your jaw muscles for 10-15 seconds. Alternate until you feel better.

If you are one of the millions who suffer from jaw pain and teeth grinding, you will instantly know the relief that comes when it ends. The body is very complex in that everything is highly connected. Grinding your teeth leads to broken teeth, neck pain, shoulder pain, facial stiffness, etc. When you take the time to care for yourself and relieve the source of tension, then the pain lifts. It can be as simple as that.

Relief for Teeth Grinding and Jaw Tension

- Ask your spouse or partner, if you have one, if they **hear you grinding** or clicking your teeth at night.

- **Check the tension levels in your face and jaw when you awaken.** If they are tense, massage them starting back at the point where your jaw comes together near your ears. Decreasing that tension first thing in the morning can prevent some headaches later on.

- **Visit your dentist** to see if he or she can spot signs of tooth grinding. They may want to fit you for a mouthguard.

- Get a massage from someone who specializes in **trigger point myotherapy or cranial sacral work**. They can release key points of pressure for surprising relief.

- Relax your teeth and jaw before bed using any of the techniques on previous pages; warm washcloths on the face, Belladonna, etc. Always consult your physician before trying new medication.

- **Don't check your email, Blackberry® or Iphone® before bed!** It reminds you of work and it increases your stress when you want it the least.

- Investigate a the **mouthguard treatment called NTI**. www.nti-tss.com

- I use Plackers *Grind No More* at night, which are lightweight, small teeth protectors. Much more comfortable than a regular mouthguard, these are disposable after a few days. I let mine soak in water and hydrogen peroxide.

Instant Stress Reliever # 2 Sleep
Lack of It Can Cause Strokes and Cancer

"Without enough sleep, we all become tall two-year-olds."
JoJo Jensen

In today's busy, hurry up world, more people are finding they have less time to get everything done. The challenge of managing multiple priorities weighs heavily, especially on entrepreneurs. 13% of those polled by *Fortune Small Business* reported having trouble getting to sleep *every* night. So what do we do? All too often, we sacrifice precious sleep, which is quite dangerous.

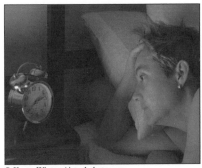

© Karen Winton / istockphoto.com

A 2014 study in the *Neurobiology of Aging* shows that lack of sleep can cause brain damage and shrinkage, and may accelerate the onset of Alzheimer's.[1] According to *Forbes*, if you get less than 7 hours of sleep, you are at a "cognitive disadvantage;" your brain does not function properly. You probably have noticed this yourself, when you awaken groggy and can't quite seem to focus. People who get less than 7 hours of sleep are 3 times more susceptible to colds, because they are suppressing their immune system. People who sleep less than 6 hours a night **quadruple** their risk of stroke, according to a University of Alabama study. **Lack of sleep is a major cause of obesity and diabetes.** Those who sleep between 7 and 8.9 hours a night on average have healthy weights; those with less do not. [2] Another study found that after three nights of interrupted sleep, otherwise healthy people require more insulin to process the glucose in their food. This effect is equivalent to gaining 20 pounds! [3] And the World Health Organization is considering labeling lack of sleep (less than 7 hours) a carcinogen (cancer causing agent.) [4] **So actually getting less than 7 hours of shuteye could cause cancer.** The current statistics are grim. 40% of the US population gets less than 7 hours a night.[5] 70 million Americans suffer from sleep problems, according to Dr. Dan Naim.[6] Are you one of them?

Consider this story of Cynthia McKay, CEO of Le Gourmet Gift Basket, of CO.

⏱ *Cynthia got very little sleep, mostly because her mind raced with ideas "due to the stress of business ownership and jet lag," she said. While her company experienced significant growth in other countries like Australia and Canada, she struggled to keep up with the pressure and lack of sleep. One day it truly cost her. Restless all night, she finally dozed at dawn, only to discover to her horror that she had missed her flight to Australia, where she was scheduled to train 17 new employees. Unable to catch a flight until the next day, McKay realized that her new employees were doing nothing but waiting for her, costing her thousands of dollars in food and hotel expenses. "It was an expensive mistake." That wake-up call led her to change her life. She now does Pilates workouts regularly, spends time with her dog, and stops consuming caffeine after 11 AM. She uses power naps throughout the day to stay fresh.*[7]

The Frequency of Insomnia

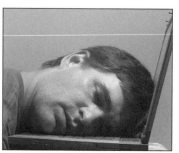

© imbarney22 / istockphoto.com

Duke University found that more than 50% of adults have insomnia at least a few times a week.[8] A study at the University of Chicago Medical Center says **an extra hour of sleep a day could reduce your chance of heart attack** as you age. Fewer than 5 hours of sleep a night leads to coronary artery calcification, which is a marker of heart disease. Insomniacs produce high levels of cortisol, which increases stress, so it is a vicious cycle.[9] 2014 research from Great Britain shows that poor sleep was the strongest predictor of pain for people over age 50. Lack of sleep creates more pain in the body.[10]

Sleep loss is quite hazardous. **Staying awake for 24 straight hours is equivalent to having blood alcohol levels of .10% - beyond the legal limit**

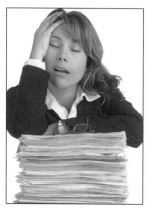

© DNY59 / istockphoto.com

for driving in the US.[11] Many of us have seen drivers weave across a highway; they may not be drunk, they may be sleep-deprived. Some of the world's worst accidents are related to inadequate sleep: Chernobyl and Three Mile Island.

Consider Naps

Naps of half an hour or less do not interfere with sleep patterns, and they can restore clarity, alertness, and memory. Edison, Einstein, and Churchill were all nappers.[12] Zappos.com, a creative and profitable on-line shoe business, has a nap room and employees are encouraged to use it regularly. Ben and Jerry's has a nap room, as do many railroads. *"What other 26-minute investment gives you a 54% productivity boost?"* asks Mark Rosekind. A consultant at Alertness Solutions in CA, he conducted sleep research at Stanford University. At Brightidea.com, employees are encouraged to nap at the office. They often wake up with great new ideas. The CEO says, *"I'd rather have employees rested and ready to handle a new challenge."* [13] At Yarde Metals of Pelham, NH, the nap room is a soundproof space with a dimmer switch and sofa. A Harvard study showed a 30-minute nap improved the performance of workers, re-establishing their productivity levels to start of the day energy. [14]

I personally am a big fan of naps, particularly late in the day when my energy is fading. I find that a short nap gives me great energy for another 6 or 7 hours. And I am not alone. 37 percent of Americans nap at least once a week. Over 1/3 say their company actually permits napping during breaks, with 16 % providing a place to nap.

Sara Mednick, author of *Take a Nap, Change Your Life*, says a 20 minute power nap is stage two sleep, very light and easy to wake from, and good for your motor memory. A nap of 20 - 60 minutes is slow wave sleep, which is quite restorative. It promotes muscle growth, tissue growth, as well as memory performance.

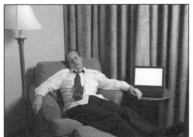
© tapshooter / istockphoto.com

"Sleepiness alone costs the American economy and employers about 18 billion dollars a year," says Darrel Drobnich of the National Sleep Foundation in Washington, DC. So why not address that proactively and provide a nap space at work?

The Positive Impact of Naps

Here's why naps are so good for you. They:
• sharpen memory
• restore clarity, alertness and good mood
• improve performance for athletes and professionals, alike.
Remember that naps from 20- 30 minutes are most effective, and you'll sleep better in the dark with a light blanket.

So consider your work schedule, suggest HR implement a nap room at your workplace, or if you work at home, set up a nap time that works around the kids and your energy level. Naps are one way to get more sleep, and according to research worldwide, we all could use more of that.

Remember- Lack of Sleep is Dangerous

Lack of sleep has so many negative outcomes. It:

• increases the risk of getting cancer, especially breast and prostate cancer
• causes brain shrinkage, brain damage and may contribute to Alzheimers
• contributes to weight gain, diabetes and obesity
• lowers the immune system function and increases the risk of infection
• causes depression and irritability, as well as feeling out of control
• damages and prematurely ages skin through excess cortisol production
• dramatically increases the risk of stroke
• contributes to pain and fibromyalgia in people over age 50 [15]

Instant Stress Relief For Those Who Have Trouble Sleeping

• Consider listening to **a noise machine** with ocean sounds, waterfalls, nature sounds. Brookstone, Target, and Walmart carry several models. Most smart phones have apps for that. I use 'White Noise'™ on my iphone®.

• **Establish a healthy bedtime routine**. Go to bed at the same time every night. Prepare your bedroom: no tv, computers, or phones. If you must have a phone in your bedroom, put it at least 3 feet away from your head, to protect you from radiation and EMF. Create a quiet, **very dark** space that is cool.[16]

• **Stop drinking caffeine after 11 AM**. That means no sodas as well.

• **Do NOT check your email before bed**. You just increase your chances of stress and tossing and turning. **Stop looking at a computer screen or phone screen at least 1 hour before bed**, because the blue light wavelength will upset your sleep patterns. Be sure your alarm clock has red light not blue light.[17]

• **Take a warm bath before bed**. Try using jasmine scented bath oil, as jasmine is said to promote better sleep. So is lavender.

• If your spouse snores, get them **a snore device**, like BreatheRight® strips.

"A good laugh and a long sleep are the best cures in the doctor's book."
Irish Proverb

"The best bridge between despair and hope is a good night's sleep."
E. Joseph Cossman

Instant Stress Reliever # 3 Eat the *Right* Food
It Can Truly Make a Difference!

"Eating is not merely a material pleasure. Eating well gives a spectacular joy to life and contributes immensely to goodwill and happy companionship. It is of great importance to the morale."
Elsa Schiaparelli

Overeating as a Result of Stress

When you're upset or depressed, what do you do? Go for a run, call a friend, or open the refrigerator? All too many people start eating and this is one key factor in the worldwide obesity epidemic. Obesity is *directly* linked to stress. The World Health Organization writes: *"Obesity has reached epidemic proportions globally, with more than 1 billion adults overweight."*[1] An Australian study showed that the body actually releases a molecule when under stress which causes fat cells to multiply and expand.[2] *That means stress itself causes fat to expand*!!!! That is startling data and it has huge implications for controlling obesity and staying healthy.

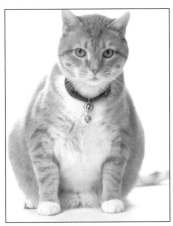

© cydebergerac / istockphoto.com

Nearly 50% of US dogs and cats are obese, straining their bodies and promoting disease.[3] Serve them healthy food at set times, play with them, and get them to run.

Here's Crystal Smith's story:

"Stress has always equaled 'snack' for me. It's best that I don't snack at all — one cookie could very well end up being a whole package. The last time it happened ...was toward the end of a long court battle over a family member's estate. I was overwhelmed, and I had just had it. I found myself with a cup of ice cream, some cookies, just nibbling." [4]

Crystal became aware of her unhealthy snacking, and with guidance and a new program, she switched to fruit and exercise and has lost 30 pounds! You can do the same thing.

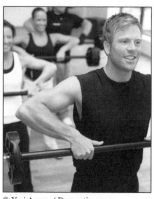

Much of the rise in obesity is due to an increased intake of foods high in saturated fats and sugars, which also contribute to diabetes. By monitoring and changing your eating habits like Crystal did, and by adopting a more physically active lifestyle, you can reduce your stress and lose weight. It's all your choice.

© Yuri Arcurs / Dreamstime.com

"Your choices today determine your tomorrow and you make your life through the power of choice."
Kathy Smith

🕐 *Belly fat can be annoying but for Stephane Gouin, a 35-year-old computer analyst, it was downright dangerous. His bulge meant excess visceral fat around his liver. Visceral fat releases toxins in the body and increases cholesterol, blood pressure and the risks of diabetes and hypertension. To his credit, Stephane took action. He shifted his five soda a day and fast food diet for meals rich in high fiber. Using weight-training and cardio workouts, he lost 35 pounds in less than nine months. He's also built muscle and strength with a home gym. All of his hard work has paid off: his resting heart rate has dropped to 68 BPM, and his blood pressure is down from 120/85 to 106/64.*[5] If Stephane can do it, you can, too.* **Note: Consult your physician and nutritionist before making any changes to your normal routine or changing medication. The author does not claim to have any medical expertise.**

Surprising Foods Which Promote Greater Health

When stress hormones like cortisone zap your body, over 1400 chemical changes occur. Stress creates deficiencies throughout your body and chemical system, causing your immune system to be depleted and triggering problems such as insomnia, poor diet, headaches, backaches, and worse. One of the easiest ways to treat stress is by eating the right food.

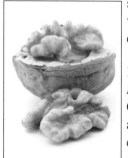

© vosmanius / istockphoto.com

1. Eat walnuts to treat depression. *Harvard Science Review* published a study by McClean Behavioral Genetics Laboratory citing that walnuts are powerful antidepressants! What a surprise: a healthy way to beat depression. If you don't like walnuts, try molasses or sugar beets instead. They have the same benefits.[6] Always consult your doctor.

2. **Eat more fish to prevent depression and feel optimistic!** Omega 3 oils in fish or fish supplements cut the risk of depression by 50%! Two or more servings a week can halve your risk of stomach, colon and pancreatic cancer.[7] Try eating wild caught salmon a few times a week. Be careful of too much tuna, since it often has high mercury.

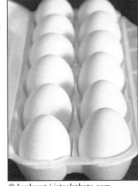

3. **Consume eggs.** 38% of women who experience depression have low folic acid. Eggs are a great source of folic acid. Eggs *"contain the highest-quality food protein known to mankind....egg protein is often the standard by which all other proteins are judged,"* says dietitian Carolyn Snyder of the Cleveland Clinic. Other sources of folic acid are leafy greens, peas and papayas.[8]

4. **Eat cauliflower, broccoli, cabbage or kale** to replenish stress-relieving B vitamins, including

© kenhurst / istockphoto.com

pantothenic acid. This acid helps turn carbohydrates and fats into usable energy and improves your ability to respond to stress by supporting your adrenal glands.[9] If you are tired, experience numbness, tingling or burning pain in the feet, you may need more B vitamins. Check with your doctor. And remember that baked potatoes are rich in Vitamin B6, which helps lower your risk of depression, according to a Brigham Young University study.

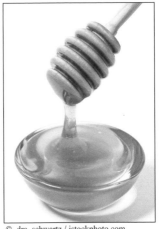

5. **Honey is very good for you**, since it makes a natural antibacterial agent. Many countries use it medicinally to treat burns and wounds, and in the United States, it has been proven to be effective in treating stress, diabetes, Alzheimer's and osteoporosis.[10]

As a professional speaker, I find that honey is wonderful to consume before a speech, as it coats the throat. It also helps zap away a sore throat when you might be getting a cold. Try it in a cup of hot water with a little bit of lemon.

© dra_schwartz / istockphoto.com

6. **Hot sauce triggers your endorphins** and lifts your spirits, says University of PA psychologist Paul Rozen.

7. **Skip the sugar and sugar substitutes**. Sugar has been linked to many different kinds of illness, and emotionally, it contributes to mood swings and drops

in energy. It also is a major factor in weight gain. If you want to learn how truly destructive sugar is, read the book *Sugar Blues* by William Dufty. Sugar substitutes have been reported to damage the kidney and liver. There are natural alternatives which sweeten your food.

🕐 *If you have a big sweet tooth, as I do, try using the herb stevia, which has no calories and no side effects. It tastes great and works just like sugar to sweeten anything. I've used it for over a decade and put it into homemade whipped cream and various dessert recipes. I carry packets with me in my purse. You can find many varieties at the store. Check to make sure they have nothing else added. I like the brand Stevita™.*

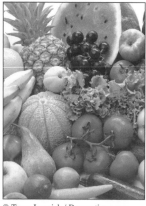

© Tomo Jesenick / Dreamstimescom

8. **Eat 5-8 servings a day of fruits and vegetables.** We've all heard this, but here's why it's true: they are chock full of antioxidants, vitamins and fiber. Vitamin C has been shown to lower blood pressure and help cortisol levels return to normal. Mix it up - try to eat several different colored fruit and veggies a day! **Blackberries have more than double the amounts of vitamin C, calcium and magnesium than blueberries.** Both boost your memory and are great for you! Choose organic ones to prevent pesticide ingestion.

🕐 *My husband and I started an organic container garden years ago. We grow fresh lettuce, cherry tomatoes, cucumbers and more. There is nothing like the flavor of fresh picked vegetables! And if you're too busy, try picking up local produce at a farm stand, farmer's market or farm co-op. The fresher and the more local the food, the better and healthier for you.*

9. Sprinkle your cereal or salad with **wheat bran** to cut your anxiety levels. Wheat bran ups your levels of GABA, an amino acid which calms the nervous system area connected to anxiety.[11]

10. **Eat pistachio nuts** to cut inflammation, lower cholesterol levels, and improve your body's response to stress. Just 1.5 ounces of pistachios provides a boost of energy and can slow the absorption of carbohydrates in the body when eaten together. One reason pistachios are so good for you is that they have large amounts of potassium.

11. **Eating kiwi fruit** can boost your immunity. A recent New Zealand study shows it reduces inflammation, and balances bacteria in the digestive system.

12. **Eat good mood foods**. Serotonin is the neurotransmitter which helps us feel good and lifts our spirits. Good sources of serotonin are sunflower seeds, mangoes, bananas, turkey, broccoli and avocados.[12]

13. Have a cup of tea, especially green or white tea, several times a day. Drinking tea reduces stress and cortisol levels. Green tea is full of "catechin polyphenols" with high levels of antioxidants. Japanese women who drink lots of green tea live longer.[13] Tea improves your concentration and prevents bone loss. A University of London study states one cup of tea can significantly reduce anxiety levels after suffering an upset.[14] An Australian study showed that drinking tea can reducing the chance of developing Type 2 diabetes by 1/5. Just be sure not

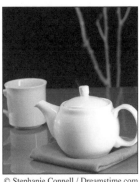

© Stephanie Connell / Dreamstime.com

to have cream or lemon in your tea, as they seem to lessen its positive impact. Take some time for yourself and have a tea break instead of a coffee break; you'll relax *and* be healthier.

14. Here's one most women already know- **eat chocolate, especially dark chocolate** (in moderation, of course!) A very potent endorphin-producing food, chocolate has 300 different compounds which activate various centers in your

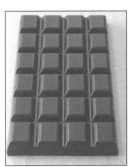

brain. Many studies have shown that it reduces stress and helps recovery from heart attacks. A study in Toronto says that eating chocolate once a week significantly lowers the risk of stroke.[15] A German study in the *European Heart Journal* showed that eating dark chocolate (1/4 of an ounce day) had lowered blood pressure and reduced the risk of heart attack by 39%. Another study found that eating dark chocolate daily reduced the levels of the stress hormone cortisol.[16] The flavinoids in dark chocolate protect damage to blood vessels that

© Maja Schon / Dreamstime.com   can lead to stroke. The best variety to reduce stress is dark chocolate with at least 70% cocoa content.

15. Be conscious of your eating habits and life choices. Consider this story of a friend of mine, whose difficult life circumstances led to obesity and cancer.

Ⓛ *Just a few short years ago, Andrea [not her real name] weighed over 400 pounds. Not a tall woman, her obesity led to significant health challenges. She was often frustrated with lack of understanding and compassion from her doctors. They expected her to have the usual medical complications from obesity: lack of energy, shortness of breath, predisposition to diabetes. What they did not expect was her cancer, and they almost missed it. Initially she had pain and discomfort in her abdomen; her doctors* *discounted her aches and pains. But finally, after the pain persisted, they did exploratory surgery, and discovered awful news: **she had cervical cancer**. A few weeks later, she started hemorrhaging and had to have both her cervix and uterus removed, as doctors rebuilt her pelvic floor. With typical good humor, she said, "Now I have a pergo and formica pelvic floor!"*

*What was most difficult for this woman is that while recovering with an open wound and 178 staples in her body, her husband was out partying until 2 AM. (His way of coping with her cancer.) She needed his help to go to the bathroom and often, he was not there. One sad morning, she courageously confronted him and said, **"If you can't be here to support me through this, I don't want to be married to you anymore."** So on top of nearly dying from cervical cancer, coping with obesity and recovery from surgery, she added the heartbreaking stress of divorce from a husband of 20 years. In spite of her agony, she still hostessed a Christmas party at her home for her co-workers ten days later, saying she needed to focus on good things and good people. Preparing for the party gave her hope.*

*How did this strong, resilient woman cope with two devastating events in her life and keep going? Good friends, a great attitude, laughter and gratitude for her blessings all lifted her spirits. Funny things, balloons and Sesame Street characters helped. Dave Sederis' books delighted her. She recovered fully and was in complete remission for seven years. She later married a wonderful man who cherishes her. **She took the lessons from her cancer into all areas of her life and began to enjoy each day more fully**. Three years ago, a small tumor had to be removed and last year, she had a lumpectomy from her breast. Her doctors are optimistic about her health and longevity. Relative to her obesity, she exercises regularly and continues to lose weight in a healthy manner. To date, she has lost over 110 pounds and keeps going. Using a variety of stress relieving techniques from exercise, physical therapy, massage, and scheduled play time, she takes great care of herself. She has eliminated all sugar from her diet, eats right and thrives with a fabulous attitude. What she learned most from all of these life-threatening experiences is that she had to make a commitment to herself to do whatever it took to stay alive and healthy, because **she wants to live.***

You can make the same commitment to *live* with less stress in your life. No matter what your challenges, you can choose to take action right now to be healthier. You can eat foods that cut your stress, exercise more often and in ways that are fun for you, prevent obesity, diabetes and cancer. It's all up to you. What's your choice?

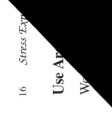
Instant Stress Reliever # 4 Aromatherapy
When Life Hands You Lemons,
Take Them to Work

"The fragrance always stays in the hand that gives the rose."
George William Curtis

Believe it or not, the scent of lemon in the workplace cuts keyboard mistakes by 50%![1] It's true. And while keyboard mistakes are not a huge source of stress, they can lead to major problems when the wrong data is put into a contract, or the wrong digit is typed into a mortgage agreement. (Our new neighbors just received their closing documents with a plot plan for a home in a completely different city!) The scent of lemons also creates a greater sense of altruism and generosity, so they could enhance your home or work life.[2]

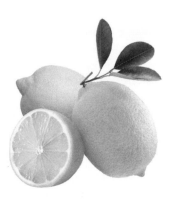

© Valentyn75 / Dreamstime.com

Fragrance is powerful

Realtors know this well. They often put drops of cinnamon oil on lightbulbs when showing a house, or bake cookies with cinnamon in them. The scent of cinnamon is said to be the most soothing and welcoming for many Americans because it reminds them of breakfast with grandparents and cinnamon toast.

Have you ever noticed how certain scents are linked to powerful memories? *I grew up in a sad household, where my mother was dying. To cope with my life challenges, I spent as much time outside as possible. My favorite place as a little girl was my grandmother's rose garden. She had dozens of brightly colored flowers which smelled heavenly. After a while, just the scent of roses soothed me and lifted my spirits. I did not know then that roses are said to promote balance and a sense of security, but they certainly worked for me. To this day, rose is still my favorite fragrance. Which scents evoke happy childhood memories for you?*

omatherapy to Treat Stress

rldwide, aromatherapy or smelling certain essential oils from plants, has been used to help treat chronic pain, insomnia, depression and stress. Aromatherapy has been used for over 6000 years. The Chinese burned scented incense to enhance harmony and balance. Ancient Greeks and Romans used essential oils for healing and promoting well-being. They all understood the healing properties of fragrance.

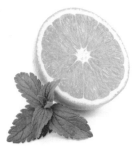

© SednevaAnna / istockphoto.com

So how does aromatherapy work? It's simple. You sniff a specific scent, through a flower, a piece of cinnamon toast or through an oil, a candle, incense or airspray. Inhaling the fragrance has various results. The scents of peppermint, cinnamon, orange or rose revitalize you while lavender, marjoram and sandalwood relax you. **Peppermint extract** on your forehead or temples can help relieve pain immediately. It's also great for concentration. A University of Cincinnati study found that people who breathe in peppermint oil are immediately more alert and better able to focus. Children who eat a peppermint before tests score better. Athletes who inhale peppermint scent have more energy. Try it the next time you work out.

Lavender oil has many uses, from relaxation to curing headaches. Because its two main compounds soothe the nervous system, your body is able to relax and have less blood vessel constriction, which causes headache pain.[3] Lavender

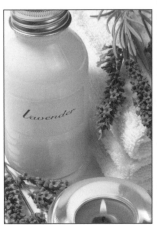

calms irritability, soothes tension and promotes relaxation. You'll notice that some fine hotels now have lavender eyemasks in their sleep kits. **Mango** is also a wonderful sleep inducer. Try mango-scented body lotion before bed.

Jasmine reduces anxiety and boosts happiness, according to a Rutgers University study. Try a jasmine scented candle.[4]

Vanilla oil is a refreshing way to soothe restless children. It has a positive impact on the limbic center of the brain, which controls emotion, according to a study done at Sloan Kettering

© Togoshi / istockphoto.com

Cancer Center in NY. A few drops on the wrists of a child can transform a cranky, whiny child into one who is happy and laughing. Try this on your next road trip.[5]

Evergreen scents like pine and spruce are powerful energizers, which revitalize you. The fragrance actually stimulates the reticular activating system in the brain, the part that relates to alertness. It works instantly, so you might want some evergreen candles or spray handy for a quick whiff. Need your work team or sports team to be more supportive of each other? Want to create better camaraderie? Try the scent of **eucalyptus**.

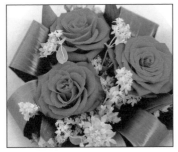

© Valeria Titoval / Dreamstime.com

According to recent research by Dr. Alan Hirsch, the fragrance raises empathy by 19%, enabling you to see things from another's point of view. Eucalyptus stimulates the beta waves at the front of the brain, promoting understanding and compassion.[6]

Work with lots of women in your office? Women who receive flowers unexpectedly are happier, even three days later. Whether it's from fragrance or the visual impact, women with flowers around experience less anxiety and have more innovative ideas at work.[7] That's true whether the flowers were sent to them or not! So if there are plenty of females at your workplace, you might want to bring in a bouquet!

How to Get More Fragrance Stress Relief in Your Life

- To bring lemons into the workplace, try **lemon-scented air fresheners**, lemon-scented candles, scent diffusers, lemon oils or lemonade.

- Spend some time reflecting on your favorite childhood memories. Which scents are associated with them? Once you remember, you can incorporate that scent in your home or workspace with perfumes, essential oils or candles.

- Go into a candle store or essential oil store and take a whiff of various fragrances and note your reaction to them. Some you will love, others you will abhor. Observe what kind of reaction each evokes in you and choose the scents accordingly.

- **Keep peppermints or peppermint oil on hand** before a challenging assignment or to give to your kids before school. Have some vanilla oil in the car for long road trips.

- There are all sorts of scent diffusers now in long sticks in lovely bottles with scent. Find one that has the right fragrance for you.

- Read some books and articles on aromatherapy.

Instant Stress Reliever # 5 Water
One of the Most Vital & Overlooked Keys to Stress Reduction

"If there is magic on this planet, it is contained in water."
Loran Eisely

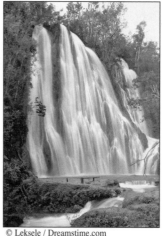

© Leksele / Dreamstime.com

Did you know that we start out our life as 99% water, before we are born? By adulthood, we are 70% water and when we die, we are close to 50% water. Blood is 92% water, bones are 22% water and muscles are 75% water.[1] As Masaru Emoto writes, *"We exist mostly as water."*[2]

Every cell in our body depends on water to function properly. Throughout our day, we lose about 10 cups of water, which must be replenished. A 5% drop in body fluids will cause a 25-30% loss in energy; a 15% drop causes death. It is estimated that 80% of North Americans are suffering from dehydration, which results in:

- energy loss and fatigue
- mental and physical exhaustion
- asthma and allergies because of restricted airways
- headaches and stiff joints because of weakened cartilage
- dry mouth, eyes, and sinuses
- sleep disturbance
- anxiety, stress and premature aging
- overeating (because people who are hungry are usually thirsty first)
- high cholesterol
- bladder problems and kidney stones
- digestive issues
- cancer and diabetes.[3 and 4]

Can you see now why the old adage, *"drink 8 glasses of water a day,"* is more important than ever? In fact, some doctors recommend 9 glasses for women and 12 glasses a day for men. [5] Often overlooked, water is vital to health, to life and to stress reduction.

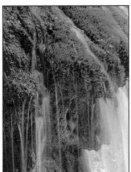

"The human body produces pain and develops various diseases when it is suffering from drought."
Fereydoon Batmanghelidj, M.D

© Irochka | Dreamstime.com

🕐 *Blogger David Seah was experiencing some significant back pain where it seemed that "each vertebra were crunching against each other like little disks of sand." Doing some research, he eventually discovered that a **common cause of joint and back pain is dehydration!** After further study and drinking large quantities of water, in 12 hours, David felt dramatically better.* [6]

Instant Stress Relief from the Water in Nature

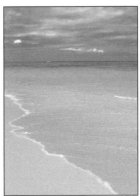

Did you know that waterfalls and oceans produce negative ions, electron-packed molecules, which calm and soothe you? Spend some time at either one of these beautiful spots and observe how much better you feel. Just 15-30 minutes can relieve depression. If you aren't near one, try running through a sprinkler or standing next to a splashing fountain for the same benefits.[7]

© Dhoxax / shutterstock.com

🕐 *For me, nothing beats the ocean; it's where I let go of stress. Walking along the beach has always soothed me and now I know why. Those negative ions bombard me and erase the negativity. I always feel better - always. The same is true of waterfalls. I find them to be refreshing and revitalizing. Try either one yourself and watch your stress melt away. Just listening to the rhythmic sound of crashing waves or rushing water can relieve tension. Listen to a CD or wave machine for a break.*

Baths are also terrific stress relievers. They can relieve joint pain, muscle stiffness and a host of other problems. The heat dilates your blood vessels and relaxes everything. It also quiets the adrenal system, reducing the fight or flight syndrome associated with severe stress.[8] Baths also help you sleep. A study from the *Journal of Physiological Anthropology* found that women who took either a 20 minute bath or soaked their legs up to their knees in hot water for 30 minutes slept better than those who did neither. If you don't have time for a bath, try running warm water on your wrists.[9]

Water as a Potent Energy Field

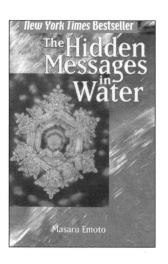

If you saw the movie *"What the Bleep Do We Know?"* about quantum physics and the power of thought, you are already familiar with the incredible research of Dr. Masaru Emoto. Science has long known that the physical world is impacted by energetic fields. Quantum physics explores that relationship in depth.

Dr. Emoto approached his research very scientifically. As surprising as it sounds, he has proven after 20 years of research that our thoughts and emotions dramatically affect water. By conducting hundreds of experiments with words put on water bottles and thoughts sent to the water, he used high speed photography to capture images of frozen water crystals. If the words were *"Love and Gratitude,"* the most exquisitely beautiful crystal formed. If the words were *"You make me sick; I will kill you,"* the crystal had tortured and ugly distortions. The same was true of classical music versus acid rock. The acid rock created ugly, harsh crystals. Experiment after experiment proved the same lesson: w*hen positive, grateful, loving thoughts were sent to the water, beauty resulted.* Hateful, negative and angry thoughts created ugliness and distortion. Pretty amazing research, humm? It certainly gives us pause and something to consider.

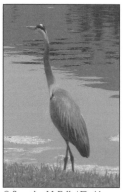

© Snowden McFall / Florida

How Our Thoughts Can Heal Water

Taking his research further, Dr. Emoto has continued to learn some extraordinary things. While it may defy traditional thinking, quantum physics supports much of his theory. Today, a great deal of Dr. Emoto's work focuses on world peace. A few years ago, he participated in an extraordinary event at a polluted lake in Japan, Lake Biwa. A group of 350 people gathered around the lake and focused on world peace. They just held the thought of "world peace," and some chanted it. That's all. A month later, a miracle occurred. **The putrid algae which had contaminated the lake and caused the awful stench did not appear that year!** Dr. Emoto says that the energetic vibration sent to water made the difference, just as it has in all the water bottle experiments.[10] **The implications of this research are profound.** If this data can be replicated again and again, it means each of us can influence the health of water on the planet.

How to Get More Stress Relief with Water

- Avoid drinking soda. The active ingredient is phosphoric acid, which leaches calcium from your bones, causing osteoporosis.

- Don't drink your water as coffee, tea or soda with caffeine. Caffeine acts as a diuretic, so you need 2 cups of water for every cup of caffeine you consume.

- Drink at least 9 glasses of purified water a day. Reverse osmosis water is best, since it removes all toxins and impurities.

- Don't drink water out of plastic bottles left in the sun. Singer Sheryl Crow believes this is a key reason she developed cancer, and there is growing research questioning the safety of BPA (bisphenol). A 2007 report titled "*Bottled Water Myths: Separating Fact from Fiction*," published in the journal Practical Gastroenterology, warns of the dangers of BPA, phthalates, and bacteria from bottled water. Use glass bottles instead.[11]

"We forget that the water cycle and the life cycle
are one."
Jacques Yves Cousteau

"Water is fundamental for life and health. The human right to water is indispen-
sable for leading a healthy life in human dignity.
It is a pre-requisite to the realization
of all other human rights."
The United Nations Committee on Economic, Cultural and Social Rights

Instant Stress Reliever # 6 Yoga & Exercise
Be More Flexible in Body, Mind and Spirit

"Yoga is invigoration in relaxation. Freedom in routine. Confidence through self control. Energy within and energy without."
Ymber Delecto

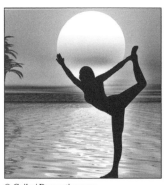
© Guilu / Dreamstime.com

Exercise Reduces Stress

According to the former US Surgeon General, C. Everett Koop, 60% of all Americans do not get sufficient exercise to strengthen their own immune system. Exercise helps release "feel-good" hormones like serotonin, beta-endorphin, and dopamine into your system. According to Tufts Health & Nutrition Letter, even a "sometimes workout" can reduce the risk of heart failure by 18%. The authors of *Younger Next Year* claim that 70% of what you *feel* as aging is optional, if people would exercise seriously one hour a day, six days a week.

The key to exercise is to make it fun; get an exercise buddy, or take a yoga or dance class. Even modest exercise like standing an extra 30 minutes a day can add three years to your life! Sitting all day is becoming increasingly detrimental to health, increasing inflammation, contributing to cancer, diabetes and stroke. A new wave of standing and treadmill desks has been designed to curb that, and I use one myself, with great results.

A Powerful and Positive Form of Exercise: Yoga

Practiced for over 5000 years, yoga is a profound and popular form of exercise, with nearly 11 million Americans practicing it.[1] It's taught around the world in many different forms. Studies at the University of NC Hospitals and Duke University show yoga reduces stress and also provides significant improvements for those with illnesses such as arthritis, back pain, cancer, diabetes, epilepsy, etc. It has even been shown to help breast cancer and menopausal patients find relief from symptoms.[2] The Center for Integrative Medicine of Thomas Jefferson University found that a 1 hour session of yoga lowered cortisol in participants with no previous yoga experience, even seven days later.[3] Practicing yoga for 20 minutes increases your focus and ability to learn, far better than aerobic exercise.[4]

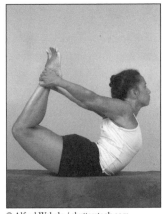

© Alfred Wakelo / shutterstock.com

The Benefits of Yoga

Whatever form of yoga you enjoy, there are enormous benefits to your body, mind and spirit. Yoga:

- increases flexibility through stretching
- improves posture and tones muscles
- promotes better breathing
- massages all internal organs of body
- increases lubrication of tendons, joints, ligaments
- flushes toxins out of the body
- reduces depression, alcoholism and PTSD in disaster survivors and war vets[5]
- provides a deep sense of relaxation and boosts moods

Yoga's stress benefits include a wide array of biochemical responses, including a decrease in the hormones produced by the adrenal glands in response to stress. Lowering levels of hormone neurotransmitters: dopamine, norepinephrine, and epinephrine creates a feeling of calm and peace.[6]

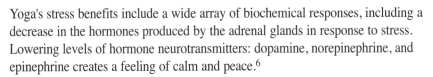

I have practiced yoga for decades and have always found it to be peaceful and relaxing. It definitely helps me be present and forget about whatever is causing me stress. My husband loves the way it opens his hips and increases his flexibility. I always feel more aligned and healthy after a yoga session, as though everything has come back into balance.

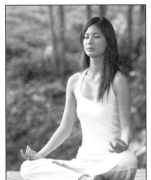

©Eastwest Imaging / Dreamstime.com

No matter what your age or ability level, you can do some form of yoga. Many corporations offer it in the office as part of their wellness program. Check it out for yourself.

Cut Your Stress Levels with Meditation

One of the common traditions at the end of yoga is a relaxation period, with closed eyes and some kind of meditation. Although it varies in each class, any kind of meditation deeply relaxes you and relieves stress.

Research validates that meditation:
- lowers blood pressure; increases circulation[7]
- improves immune function and memory
- shortens hospital stays [8]
- decreases insomnia[9]
- helps childhood stress, ADHD [10]
- helps reverse heart disease[11]

Many people wonder just how to meditate. You can start by saying a small prayer or ask inwardly that only that which is for your highest good take place. Begin deep breathing. Close your eyes, put your hand on your lower belly, and imagine filling it with breath, just like a baby does. IN = expand your belly. OUT = release belly. Fill your belly all the way up and let it out fully. Do this repeatedly, focusing on your breath.

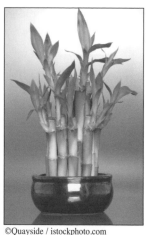

©Quayside / istockphoto.com

From here, some people imagine letting out all the bad, the toxins, frustrations, anger, etc. on their "out" breath, and breathing in love, peace, and healing on the "in" breath. Some suggest chanting a tone, like "om" pronounced "ooohhm-mm" while breathing. (It's the ancient Hindu name for God.) Some focus on a plant or a stone or some other beautiful item from nature. They contemplate that and begin to let go of the worries of the day. Others sit quietly and listen for spiritual guidance, which they may choose to write down. Mindfulness meditation has become increasingly popular. There are dozens of forms of meditation. Find a method that works for you and use it. The key is to stick with it day after day. It gets easier with time to quiet your mind and just be. And it makes a huge difference in your peacefulness and your resiliency.

I've been meditating for over twenty years with powerful results. It's how I start my day and a wonderful way to quiet down after a day's work. Everything seems to come into perspective and things I had worried about before don't seem to matter as much anymore. The deep breathing and for me, focus on God, shift me out of any limited thinking and into a more expansive place.

Both yoga and meditation may be unfamiliar to you, but they are becoming more and more mainstream, because of their impressive benefits. Consult with your doctor about which exercise practice suits you and your lifestyle best.

> *"Yoga has a sly, clever way of short-circuiting*
> *the mental patterns that cause anxiety."*
> Baxter Bell

Instant Stress Reliever # 7 Creative Expression
It Taps Into Freedom and Innocence

"To be creative means to be in love with life. You can be creative only if you love life enough that you want to enhance its beauty, you want to bring a little more music to it, a little more poetry to it, a little more dance to it."
Osho

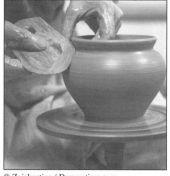

© Zojakostina / Dreamstime.com

Being Creative Keeps You in the Present

Worry is one of the typical expressions of stress and it usually involves long anguished thinking about what could go wrong in the future. A great solution is to do something creative. From coloring in a child's coloring book to writing a poem, painting a watercolor, dancing, or sculpting, creative expression is a fantastic stress reliever because **it keeps you in the present moment.** Right now, that's all there is; right this second is all you know and can participate in for sure. It's been said that the present is called that name because it is indeed a gift. You are your most receptive and your most expansive when you are here right now.

Being Creative Keeps You Young

A recent study found that a woman with a creative job has the cardiovascular fitness of someone 6 years younger! Drawing and painting improve the brain's psychological resilience, according to a 2014 German study.[1a] At Zappos.com, they interview for this trait and encourage employees to be "a little weird." They promote a fun-filled atmosphere where employees innovate great ways to satisfy customers. Examples of creative work are acting, building, singing, dancing, conducting, writing, designing, cooking, brainstorming, drawing

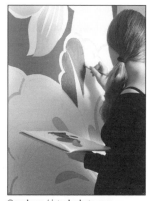

© webeye / istock photo.com

(think architects, symphony conductors, interior designers, web developers.) However, the most vital quotient is you: if you think it is exciting and interesting work where you are frequently learning, then your job has the same benefits as one in the traditionally "creative" fields.[1]

Listening to Music Can Boost Your Immune Function

A 2006 Journal of Advanced Nursing study showed that listening to music one hour a day for a week **reduced symptoms of depression by 25%.** Music, especially classical music, can also serve as a powerful stress-relief tool. Listening to Pachelbel's famous Canon in D major while preparing a public speech helps avoid anxiety and lowers heart rate and blood pressure, which usually accompany public speaking. Music therapy can also elevate mood, improve immune system function, reduce fatigue and improve self-acceptance in people. Music therapy has been shown to have beneficial health effects on cancer patients, multiple sclerosis patients, and surgical patients.[2]

🕐 *I use different CD's in the car. When I need to get Fired Up!, I have energizing, upbeat music that empowers me. When I need to relax, I listen to soft jazz and soothing instrumentals. Try this yourself, especially if you spend hours in the car each day. Make custom playlists on your MP3 player.*

Make Music with Others

Whether it's by playing instruments or singing, making music with others reinforces self-discipline and teamwork, and improves memory and health. Making music can also be an excellent tool for those with asthma, particularly learning to play wind instruments.[3] Asthmatics learn to breathe properly, to improve the function of their lungs and not to panic when an attack occurs.

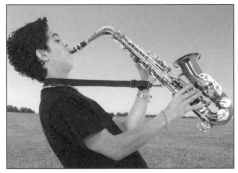
© Andres Rodriguez | Dreamstime.com

A 2005 study in *Medical Science Monitor* demonstrated that making music can reverse stress on a genomic level. 32 adults who did not consider themselves musical were subjected to a frustrating puzzle exercise designed to induce stress. One group continued to try to solve the puzzle. Another got to de-stress and read a paper or magazine. The third group played with a music-making keyboard program. The greatest amount of stress reduction came in the third group. So even if you've never made music before and don't understand music, making music can lower your stress levels.[4]

Dancing Will Cut Your Stress

According to the American Dance Therapy Association, dance is great for you physically, emotionally and mentally. It boosts your memory, because you are learning new skills, and it can reduce your risk for developing Alzheimer's by 76%. You meet new people, laugh and have fun. It's also pleasurable physical exercise and can be very romantic.[5]

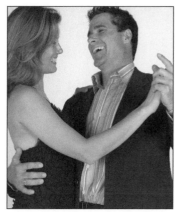

© focalhelicopter/ istockphoto.com

⏰ *My husband and I started ballroom dancing over a decade ago, and what a wonderful gift it has been. Initially, it was frustrating, because he had to learn to lead and I had to learn to follow. But as we got better and practiced more, it became a great way to work out together, and we have made many friendships with people of all ages. We try to take a class at least once a week and go dancing most weekends. Dancing for even one hour is a great stress reliever, and believe me, when you are on the dance floor, your mind cannot be anywhere else. It keeps you totally in the present moment! It's been a great source of tension relief and joy. And watching "Dancing with the Stars," or "So You Think You Can Dance," two American TV shows, only spur us to become better dancers.*

Find Your Outlet

No matter how you like to express yourself creatively, do it regularly. Whether you knit, sew, garden, dance, scrapbook, cook, woodwork, make jewelry or any one of hundreds of creative arts, lose yourself and your stress in the activity. You'll be much healthier and happier as a result.

"There is no doubt that creativity is the most important human resource of all. Without creativity, there would be no progress, and we would be forever repeating the same patterns."
Edward de Bono

Instant Stress Reliever # 8 Defuse Anger
Anger that is Unmanaged Becomes Dangerous

"When angry, count to ten before you speak. If very angry, count to one hundred."
Thomas Jefferson

Anger Can Make You Ill

Have you ever watched a young child have a really spirited temper tantrum - where they jump up and down, stomp their feet, make fists and holler? They have an emotional fit, crying and making all sorts of noise. And then ten minutes later, they're just fine. They let go of the frustration, move on and get back to being happy. Wouldn't it be nice if we adults could deal with our anger that quickly?

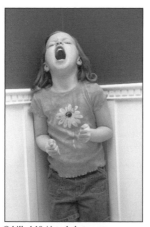

All human beings experience anger; it's a normal, healthy emotion. But when you're under stress and anger gets out of control, anger becomes destructive, to you, your relationships and your health. A 2013 German study showed that people who

© killerb10 / istockphoto.com

repressed their anger had higher cortisol levels and were 31% likelier to have high blood pressure, a heart attack, or cancer.[1a]

According to psychologist Charles Spielberger, Ph.D, anger is *"an emotional state that varies in intensity from mild irritation to intense fury and rage."* Anger triggers physiological changes in your body; your heart rate and blood pressure increase, along with the levels of your energy hormones, adrenaline, and noradrenaline. That's what creates the feelings of your heart pounding or the blood vessels in your head throbbing. You are triggering a physical reaction when you get angry.[1]

How to Deal with Your Anger

Most people deal with anger one of three ways - they express it, suppress it or calm it. Expression can be healthy, if done in a constructive manner where you strategies that have been proven successful in resolving even the most bitter conflicts. I have used it myself with great results.

If suppressed anger is not redirected, you can turn that anger on yourself, and end up depressed. The longer you suppress your anger, the more likely you are to explode at some later date, so finding healthy strategies for expressing this anger is important.[3] New research published in the Harvard Study of Adult Development states: *"workers who repress their frustration are at least three times more likely to admit that they've hit a glass ceiling in their careers. And they... have disappointing personal lives."* [4]

People who vent their anger live two years longer than those who don't according to the journal *Health Psychology.*[4a] Calming the anger through stress-relieving techniques is probably the most constructive way of dealing with anger, so long as you get it out of your system. Consider this:

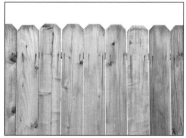

© emmgunn / istockphoto.com

🕐 *A little boy had a bad temper. His father gave him a bag of nails and told him that every time he lost his temper, he must hammer a nail into the back of the fence. The first day the boy had driven 37 nails into the fence. Over the next few weeks, as he learned to control his anger, the number of nails hammered gradually dwindled down. He discovered it was easier to hold his temper than drive those nails into the fence. Finally, the day came when the boy didn't lose his temper at all. He told his father and the father suggested the boy now pull out one nail for each day that he was able to hold his temper. The days passed and the boy was finally able to tell his father that all the nails were gone. The father took his son by the hand and led him to the fence. He said, "You have done well, my son, but look at the holes in the fence. The fence will never be the same. When you say things in anger, they leave a scar just like this one. You can put a knife in a man and draw it out. It won't matter how many times you say I'm sorry, the wound is still there." The little boy then understood how powerful his words were. He looked up at his father and said "I hope you can forgive me, Father, for the holes I put in you." "Of course I can," said the father.* [5]

Your Physiology When Angry

Your body has all sorts of physical reactions when you are angry:

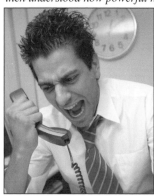

© diego cervo / istock photo.com

- your muscles tense up
- neurotransmitter chemicals surge your energy
- your heart rate increases (average heart rate of 80 climbs to 180 beats per minute)
- your breathing accelerates as you try to take in more oxygen

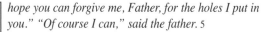

- your blood pressure soars (120 over 80 suddenly rises to 220 over 130) [6]
- your face turns red with increased blood flow
- your blood clots or coagulates, which can lead to an aneurism or blood clot
- your blood sugar drops (dangerous for diabetics or hypoglycemics)[7]

Emotions are usually intense and even if the source of your anger resolves positively, it takes a long time for your body to return to its natural resting state.

Prolonged stress and anger can lead to many health disorders: heart attacks and stroke, memory impairment, stomachaches, irritable bowel syndrome, and even vision problems, like ocular migraines, wiggly lines or light flashes (usually the result of constricted blood vessels in the brain.) [8] Chronically angry people tend to have suppressed immune systems, because of the frequent pumping in of the hormone epinephrine. According to a recent study in BMC Geriatrics, seniors who have an emotionally upsetting experience are at much greater risk of falling for the next hour after the incident.[9]

Anger in the workplace can lead to lost jobs, violence and worse. Anger at home can result in child abuse, domestic violence and broken families.[10]

Tips for Handling Anger

1. **Count to 10.** Really- try it. Just take time to simmer down and think about the consequences of losing your temper or reacting badly. What will it cost you? Is it worth it? Counting enables you to rethink your next actions.

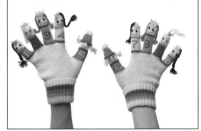

© ferrantraite / istockphoto.com

2. If you want to hit something, **hit a punching bag** at a gym or **pound pillows.** Make a stack of thick pillows and plant yourself so your legs are apart and one is behind the other by about 6 inches. Swing your arms from high over your head and pound the pillows with a loud "arrghh" or some other sound. It's very empowering! (*Yes - I have tried it myself and it helps.*)

3. **Breathe deeply at least 5 times.** Put your hands on your abdomen, fill it up all the way and let it out...slowly. Do this several times to regain control and calm your system.

4. **Take a time out.** Those of you with young children in your life know how effective this can be. When you are really upset or angry, remove yourself from

the situation, calm down, go be quiet somewhere and reflect on what you really want from the situation. Chances are good, it's not to be in conflict.

5. **Get moving.** *The Scandinavian Journal of Medicine & Science in Sports* reported that runners were 70 percent less likely to experience high stress and life dissatisfaction. Channel anger into physical movement and it will lift your spirits and be good for your physical well-being. You'd also be astonished at what a great job you do cleaning when you are angry. It can be highly satisfying to scrub pans when you're aggravated.

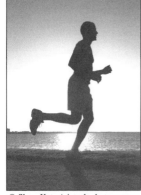

© ShaneKato / istock photo.com

6. **Use empathy.** Try to look at the situation from the perspective of the others involved. What is motivating their behavior? What's going on in their lives? It has often been said that if you walked a mile in the shoes of your enemy, you would wish them only love and good things because their life is so hard. Before you react and judge negatively, consider the other person's situation.

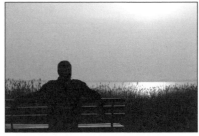

© Iryna Shpulak I Dreamstime.com

7. **Imagine you're at a peaceful place, like a favorite vacation spot.** Take a mini-vacation and change your focus from whatever is upsetting you to somewhere you find soothing and relaxing. Shift your attention and let the peaceful setting relax you.

8. **Forgive yourself and others.** This is one of the most dramatic and liberating ways to release anger. When you are very upset about what someone has done, forgiveness can be so freeing. Liberate yourself from the energy it takes to hold negative resentments or hurt feelings against someone. You don't forgive for the benefit of the other person, you forgive for yourself. The perk is that you heal your relationship and yourself. The longer you hold on to hostile feelings about someone, the more of your energy they sap. It's incredible how peaceful and calm you feel after forgiveness. In a study of over 200 subjects, Frederic Luskin, Ph.D, author of *Forgive for Good*, found that forgiveness training reduced participants' stress by 25%. Try using forgiveness as a daily practice, especially when you have judged yourself.[11]

Instant Stress Reliever # 9 Laugh
He Who Laughs, Lasts (Really!)

"I would say laughter is the best medicine, but it's more than that. Laughter brings the swelling down on our national psyche, then applies a topical antibiotic cream."
Stephen Colbert

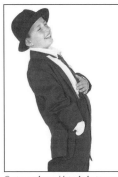

© stevecoleccs / istockphoto.com

Laughter not only makes you feel better emotionally, relieving stress and tension, but it actually helps you live longer. It's the epitome of an instant stress reliever.

Consider this story from the Internet.

Recently I received a parrot as a gift. The parrot had a bad attitude and an even worse vocabulary. Every word out of the bird's mouth was rude, obnoxious and laced with profanity. I tried and tried to change the bird's attitude by consistently saying only polite words, playing soft music and anything else I could think of to "clean up" the bird's vocabulary.

Finally, I was fed up and I yelled at the parrot. The parrot yelled back. I shook the parrot and the parrot got angrier and even ruder. So, in desperation, I threw up my hands, grabbed the bird and put him in the freezer. For a few minutes the parrot squawked and kicked and screamed. Then suddenly there was total quiet. Not a peep was heard for over a minute.

Fearing that I'd hurt the parrot, I quickly opened the door to the freezer. The parrot calmly stepped out onto my outstretched arms and said, "I believe I may have offended you with my rude language and actions. I'm sincerely remorseful for my inappropriate transgressions and I fully intend to do everything I can to correct my rude and unforgivable behavior." I was stunned at the change in the bird's attitude. As I was about to ask the parrot what had made such a dramatic change in his behavior, the bird continued, "May I ask what the turkey did?"

Now take a minute. Did you laugh? Even chuckle? Don't you feel better, even a little lighter? Laughter is great for your mind, body and spirit.

"Laughter is an instant vacation."
Milton Berle

Laughter is Very Good For You

Several studies at the University of Maryland Medical Center have demonstrated the healing power of laughter. A good hearty laugh jogs your internal organs, gives your body a workout and releases pressure. Laughter raises the level of infection-fighting T-cells, which in turn, strengthens your immune system. A recent study on diabetic patients finds that "mirthful" laughter raises good cholesterol and lowers inflammation.[1]

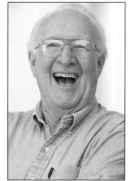
© stevecoleccs / istockphoto.com

Laughter extends your life by:
• improving your immune function
• lowering your blood pressure
• helping your heart function better
• improving your brain function [2]
• relieves pain and prevents depression.[2a]

One pioneer in laughter research, William Fry, claimed it took ten minutes on a rowing machine for his heart rate to reach the level it would after just one minute of hearty laughter. There's an instant stress reliever.[3] Another report showed that one big belly laugh is equivalent to 45 minutes of stress relief!

Laughter has even been shown to help cure terminal patients.

Norman Cousins, the author of Anatomy of an Illness, *suffered from ankylosing spondylitis, a condition that destroys collagen, which binds the body's cells together. Nearly completely paralyzed, he was given only a few months to live. He checked into a hotel and started taking large does of Vitamin C and* **laughter.** *He discovered that comedies like Marx Brothers' movies and Candid Camera shows made a huge difference in how he felt. Ten minutes of laughter allowed him two hours of pain-free sleep. Later, he returned to work full-time at the* <u>Saturday Review</u> *and lived another sixteen years.*

"Hearty laughter is a good way to jog internally
without having to go outdoors."
Norman Cousins

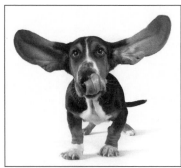

© graphicphoto / istockphoto.com

Try Laughter Clubs

So how can you get more laughter in your life? Try a Laughter Club. I'm not talking about a comedy club, although those are great, too. Believe it or not, in India, Dr. Martin Kataria started laughter clubs, where people gather to laugh for good health. Over 6000 laughter clubs exist in 60 countries around the world. There are also laughter hotlines where you can call in at various times and laugh with others.[4]

🕐 *I tried this myself and called one of the hotlines and laughed with total strangers for 20 minutes. It was a little awkward at first, but then lots of fun. I definitely felt more refreshed and relaxed afterwards. Try it when work is just too much to take.*

Dr. Lee S. Berk from Loma Linda University, California, reports that laughter increases natural killer cells (a type of white cell) and raises the antibody levels. After laughter therapy, antibodies which help protect against bacteria and viruses increase in your lungs.[5] Many members of Laughter Clubs have noticed reduced incidences of common colds, sore throats and chest infections, as well as depression and arthritis.[6]

Funny Story on the Internet - Note To Mechanic

🕐 *An auto mechanic received a repair order that read: "Check for clunking sound when going around corners." Taking the car out for a test drive, he made a right turn, and a moment later he heard a 'clunk.' He then made a left turn and again heard a 'clunk.' Back at the shop, he opened the car's trunk, and soon discovered the problem. Promptly, he returned the repair order to the service manager with the notation, "Removed bowling ball from trunk."*

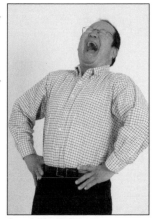

© azndc / istockphoto.com

"It is impossible for you to be angry and laugh at the same time. Anger and laughter are mutually exclusive and you have the power to choose either."
Wayne Dyer

Laughter at Work

Laughter is very important in the workplace, provided it is appropriate, tasteful and not derogatory. A recent study done in Canadian financial institutions found that the **most successful managers**, those who facilitated the highest level of employee performance, **regularly used humor at work.**

According to Thomas Kuhlman, a psychologist at the University of St. Thomas, laughter is vital when employees are in no-win situations, like having to do a job without the necessary resources of time, money, or manpower. It's also valuable when there are uncontrollable stressors, such as layoffs, crises, sudden deadlines or emergency scheduling. That makes laughter especially helpful in times like these.[7] When we have very little control over what happens to us, stress occurs. We have one choice at that time: to determine our reaction to that stress. Christoper Reeves said a few years after his disabling accident, *"The one thing I do have control over is my attitude: how I treat my caregivers."* Often the best way to cope with an impossible situation is to lighten up and laugh.

"Through humor, you can soften some of the worst blows that life delivers. And once you find laughter, no matter how painful your situation might be, you can survive it."
Bill Cosby

How to Get More Laughter in Your Life

- Listen to satellite radio; there are several comedy channels to tickle your funnybone. Be careful; some are X-rated!

- Spend time with a young child- they laugh often, as much as 400 times a day and most adults laugh 10 or fewer times.

- Watch comedy TV shows: Stephen Colbert, Jay Leno, Dave Letterman, Jon Stewart or old Nick at Nite sitcoms. (I'm a big fan of *Friends* reruns.)

- Listen to comedy CD's, podcasts or mp3's from comics like Bill Cosby, Jeff Foxworthy, or Ellen DeGeneres.

- Read *Readers Digest* funny stories.

- Go to www.youtube.com and search for funny videos.

- Collect funny movies and videos, whatever is funny to you.

- Read funny books, daily comics or cartoon books.

- Ask your friends: "What's the funniest thing that has happened to you?"

Instant Stress Reliever # 10
Spend Time with Friends
It Prevents Loneliness and Increases Longevity

"A friend is a gift you give yourself."
Robert Louis Stevenson

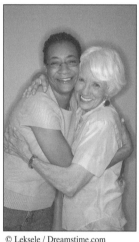

© Leksele / Dreamstime.com

Make time with friends a priority. Several years ago *Ladies Home Journal* reported many women were lonely. In 2012, more than 32 million Americans lived completely alone, with nearly 16 million being female.[1a] 20% of people feel so cut off from others that loneliness is a major source of unhappiness.[1]

The danger of the Internet world is that many of us tend to become isolated. Relationships with people online do not fulfill the deep-seeded need for human contact, touch and quality conversation. Think about it: if you have spent all day working alone on the computer, how is that filling your need for actual physical contact, hearing a friendly voice or looking into someone's warm eyes? The answer is simple - it doesn't.

Lonely people eat more fats, exercise less and are more apt to die young.[2] The stress of social isolation contributes to breast cancer susceptibility.[3] A Harvard Medical School Nurses' Health Study proports that not cultivating meaningful relationships can be as life-threatening as cigarettes.

Spending time with friends creates the release of oxytocin, a neurotransmitter that relieves stress and promotes euphoria. Those who had the most friends over a 9 year time period cut their risk of death by 60%.[4] And socializing may ward off Alzheimer's. People who socialize the most are also mentally agile: fast thinkers![5] A 2013 Dutch study showed that the more you spend time with friends, the easier it is to deal with stress.[6] A recent study in Australia showed that people in contact with at least 5 friends on a weekly basis were 22% less likely to die in 10 years.[7] A 2013 UNC study found that spending time with loved ones decreases inflammation.[8] Schedule in friend time; it could actually extend your life. It could also boost your happiness quotient. Very happy people have good relationships. Whether with a friend, partner, a parent or relative, a key indicator in two different happiness studies demonstrate that strong friendships and connections lead to joy.[9]

The Value of Friendship

"Sometimes our light goes out, but is blown again into instant flame by an encounter with another human being. Each of us owes the deepest thanks to those who have rekindled this inner light." Albert Schweitzer

Friendship is a precious gift and we never know what it will truly mean in our lives.

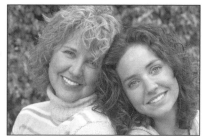

© Dana E. Fry / Shutterstock.com

ⓛ *Michelle and Kimie were close friends, who bonded even more after the awful death of Michelle's son. Michelle's only other child, a daughter, was great comfort, but Michelle needed another mom to talk to. Over the years, the two friends became like sisters. Laughing over coffee, sharing ups and downs, their friendship helped her cope. It deepened even more when Kimie was diagnosed with cervical cancer. She received aggressive treatment and the cancer went away. They celebrated, but that victory was short-lived. The cancer returned and Kimie worried how her five children would cope with moving out of town at the same time as grieving her death. She tentatively asked Michelle if she would take them in when she died. Unselfishly, Michelle promised she would. When Kimie died at age 40, Michelle and her husband took in the five kids, stretching their home and their*

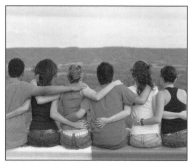

© aldomurillo / istockphoto.com

resources. Their three bedroom home was now taxed with a much bigger family and enormous grocery bills. The Orange Park, FL, Rotary Club heard what they had done and decided to help. They took out a loan and built a 1180 sq. ft. addition to the home to accommodate everyone, adding two bedrooms, two baths, a study area and laundry room. It was truly a miracle of giving that went on and on, and now everyone in that home has more love and more room! It all started because a friendship was forged.[10]

The Ripple Effect of Happiness

Happiness has a major ripple effect, impacting strangers as well as your close circle of friends. A Harvard study of over 4,000 people showed that happiness has far reaching impact, by a factor of 3. For example, if you have a happy friend who lives within one mile of you, your odds of being happy increase by 25%. A happy sibling only increases it by 14%. So your sunny friends have a stronger effect than your siblings. What was more surprising is that the happiness of a friend's friend boosts your chance of being happy by almost 10%. The effervescence of a friend of a friend of a friend

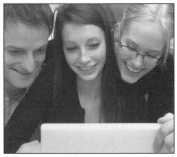

©Yuri_Arcurs / istockphoto.com

increases it by 5-6%! [11] Just think about the possibilities if you were the happy friend impacting hundreds!

Ways to Decrease Loneliness and Increase Your Happiness Quotient

Given that your happiness can impact so many other people, you owe it to yourself to change your habits, and spend more time with friends. Here are some ways to break your isolation:

• Take walks in your neighborhood and stop to chat with others. Offer to help them with various projects, like walking a dog.

• Smile at other people, like when you go to supermarkets.

• Join a volunteer organization and get to know others in the group.

Remember the Importance of Touch

While you are with your friends, remember to **get and give a hug**. Physical touch is very healing and a tremendous stress reliever. We all need touch several times a day. Hugging and kissing both signal the brain to release oxytocin, the hormone that makes you feel good and bond. Virginia Satir, a famous American psychotherapist, once said that people need 4 hugs a day to help prevent depression, 8 for psychological stability and 12 for growth. Happily married wives who held their husband's hands when shocked with electricity had lower stress response and felt less pain than when alone. Even holding a stranger's hand lowered the stress response.[10] Babies who are not touched regularly die, so touch is critical.

So as you plan your next week, schedule in time to be with friends. Give them a hug and share your joy. Make it a priority to take excellent care of the ones you have and develop new friendships as you go. It will relieve your stress, help you live longer and keep your brain sharp. Plus your happiness will ripple and help untold others, too. Don't worry - be happy!

Instant Stress Reliever # 11 Completion
The Key to Peace of Mind

"Success is how you collect your minutes.
You spend millions of minutes to reach one triumph, one moment,
then you spend maybe a thousand minutes enjoying it.
If you are unhappy through those millions of minutes,
what good are the thousands of minutes of triumph?
It doesn't equate.
Life is made up of small pleasures,
Happiness is made up of those tiny successes.
The big ones come too infrequently.
If you don't have all those zillions of tiny successes,
the big ones don't mean anything."
Norman Lear

Have you ever come home from work and wondered what you did all day? Is your TO DO list never-ending with very little getting crossed off? Frustrating, isn't it? And exhausting. And **stressful.**

Completion is Essential

Incompletions drain large amounts of energy and actually create stress. Anything from half-read books to cluttered closets to the classic "to do" lists that never get finished; these are all incompletions. Incompletions are a form of self-sabotage which can create anxiety, worry and tension. Researchers at UCLA found that just looking at clutter creates more production of the stress hormone cortisol.[1] Clutter and incompletions pile up, creating anxiety. Every day, each one of us makes commitments to do things. Saying you'll be at work on time is an

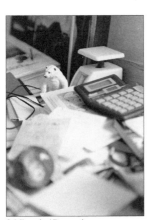

© Micropix / Dreamstime.com

agreement. Setting up lunch with a friend at a certain time and place is an agreement. Promising to take out the garbage tonight is an agreement. Most people are good at keeping agreements with others. People who don't keep agreements don't have many friends, because they aren't trust-worthy. *Broken agreements destroy relation-ships.* The problem for many of us is keeping agreements with ourselves. An example:

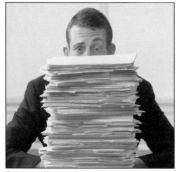

© Avava / Dreamstime.com

🕐 *Paul tells himself before going to bed that he will get up early to work out; he's starting to see a spare tire around his middle and criticizes himself for it. He sets his clock for 5:30 AM. When the alarm rings, he rolls over and goes back to sleep. What just happened? He let himself down. He has broken an agreement with himself and judges himself. If he does this enough times, he no longer will believe his own word. His self-esteem will slowly diminish and he may feel consistently tired, anxious, and frustrated with himself.*

Each incompletion is a broken agreement, and as long as something is still out there unfinished, it saps a little bit of energy. Pile up enough incompletes and you have someone who feels like a failure. Action is rewarded and inaction leads to stagnancy.

Here's Why: Completion is Powerful

In *The Path of Least Resistance*, Robert Fritz describes the circle of completion. The three phases in this circle are germination, assimilation and completion.

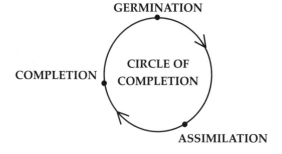

Germination is the initial start-up phase of a project. This is usually where you feel the greatest excitement and enthusiasm about your life. You'll most likely share that contagious energy with others.

Assimilation is the phase where people take action, where *you're actually doing what needs to be done to make things happen.* This is where many people get stuck and never completely finish projects. They get halfway done or they quit just short of realizing their goals. That is a big mistake because they lose out on all the joy and power that comes from **Completion**.

There is a distinct and special energy you experience every time you **complete**. Think about it. Reflect on the last time you finished some goal or project you'd been working towards for some time. How did you feel? Satisfied, pleased with yourself, perhaps even proud? That's all part of the energy of completion and that energy gets you motivated to accomplish your next goal. It actually fuels the next project.[2]

One very powerful technique is to record your successes in a journal each day. Every intention you set out to do and actually complete is a success. Whether it was to close a million dollar account or make the bed, if you set out to do it and accomplished it, to your brain, those are equal successes. (Maybe not to your emotions, but to your brain, they are!)

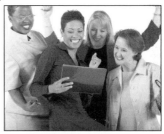

© 2009, Jupiter Images Corporation

I started doing this in my mid 20's after taking a course called "Technologies for Creating. The first year, I recorded my successes for 285 days. In December, I looked at my journal and saw I had accomplished a great deal. It made me feel successful. I observed how much I completed and my selfesteem grew. Many years later, I still do it because I am so busy with two businesses, writing books and traveling internationally that I need to feel a sense of accomplishment and give myself credit for all that I have done. It's powerful and I certainly feel different on the days I don't do it. I highly recommend it as a way to feel successful and effective.

How to Get More Completion in Your Life

• **Be very careful about your agreements**. Don't say "yes" until you are sure you can keep the commitment.[3]

• Walk through your house and notice what is incomplete. Is there a huge pile of laundry waiting to be done? Is the carpet filthy? **Take 10 minutes right now and just do it**. Feel the completion.

• Are there any **old newspapers or half-read magazines** in your home? Recycle them or throw them away.

• **Look in your closet**. Is there some article of clothing you know you will never wear again? Give it away.

• **Ask your friends**: "Is there anything I promised to do for you that I have forgotten? and then listen. If you still want to do it, make plans. If not, renegotiate the agreement.

Instant Stress Reliever # 12 Pets
Stroke a Beloved Pet- for Both of You

"A dog is the only thing on earth that will love you more than you love yourself."

Having a Pet Could Save Your Family- Literally

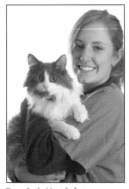

© sandocir / istockphoto.com

🕐 *Cathy, Eric and their son Michael Keesling had retired early after handling a flooded basement and setting up a gasoline pump to empty it. Their beloved mellow cat, Winnie, sat in the window enjoying the sounds of the evening. All of sudden, Michael passed out in the hallway. Cathy and Eric soon lost consciousness as well, because of a gas leak. The normally gentle Winnie sprang on Cathy, pulled her hair and yowled in her ear to wake her up. Cathy kept blacking out, but Winnie insisted. Finally, Cathy called 911 and the family was rescued. If Winnie had waited 5 more minutes, they would all be dead!"*[1]

Pets are amazing healing agents and powerful lifesavers. Trained dogs today can detect bladder cancer by sniffing urine and fire dogs can identify arsonists by smelling gasoline on their hands. Service pets save the lives of their owners every day. They can warn chronic seizure sufferers of an upcoming attack, guide the blind through a busy intersection, or provide much needed laughter and joy to hospital-bound patients. Horses have done some amazing healing work with trauma patients, just by being present, gentle and loving. Even dolphins work compassionately and effectively with disabled and sick children, giving them a new lease on life, as they well know at Dolphins Plus in Key Largo, FL.

Just Owning a Pet Reduces Your Stress

According to the the University of Minnesota's Stroke Research Center, **simply**

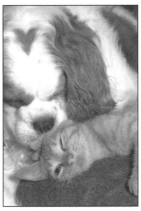

© Jeff Thrower / Shutterstock.com

owning a cat can cut the risk of heart attack. After studying subjects for 10 years, those who owned a cat were 40% less likely to die from heart attacks.[2] Other studies have demonstrated the same thing about dogs. Apparently, having pets lowers the levels of the stress hormone norepinephrine in the body, making you feel better and brightening your mood even more than being with a human friend. It might be because our pets love us unconditionally. That may be why they help us be less anxious when faced with a stressful situation.

Karen Allen, Ph.D., of the State University of New York at Buffalo, conducted a study and shares that having a non-judgmental, loving animal present is soothing to those under stress.[3]   According to WebMD, one study found that people with serious diseases like cancer are much less likely to be depressed if they have a strong tie to a pet.

Think about it in your life. If you have a pet, recall a time when you have been very anxious, upset or worried. Did you spend some time with your pet? Did you and Fido go for a walk and did he cheer you up by licking your face and making you smile? Or perhaps your cat Fluffy played "chase the fuzzy mouse" with you and helped you forget your pain. Or you went for a ride on your amazing horse and let go of the world.

⏱ *The simple act of stroking a purring cat can instantly release tension. I have had cats all my life, and one of my favorite activities at the end of the day is to cuddle up with Trinity and scratch her neck while she purrs. It immediately soothes me and releases my tension. My cat Gabriel will chirp at me when he feels I am getting too tense working on the computer. So I pick him up and cradle him like a baby; I delight in his loud purrs as he approves of my strokes. Nuzzling my cats instantly relaxes me, connects me with my heart, and helps me unwind. How about you?*

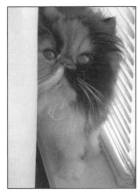

© Snowden McFall -" Trinity"

The Benefits Of Pet Ownership

• **Pets help us lower our blood pressure!** A study of hypertensive NY stock brokers who have cats or dogs as pets had lower blood pressure and lower heart rates than those who did not. When the other study members heard the test results, several in the non-pet group went out and got pets themselves! [4]

• **Pets help us be more social and more fit**. Walking a dog gets you out of your home, and tends to connect you with other people. It makes you more approachable and gives you something to share with new acquaintances.

• **Pets reduce our loneliness**. Nursing home residents were less lonely when visited by dogs than when visited by people![5]

There are hundreds of ways pets make a difference in our lives. But best of all, they are an instant, easy and loving stress reliever.

"An animal's eyes have the power to speak a great language."
Martin Buber

Get Instant Stress Relief with Pets

• If you don't have a pet, there are **wonderful shelters with free animals** to adopt. Millions are killed every year. Just be sure you can give it love, food and shelter.

• If you can't have a pet yourself, because of allergies in the home, etc. **adopt a neighbor's pet**. There are many people who are not able to get out and walk their dogs as often as they'd like, or who want their kitties to have a little more companionship.

• If you own a business, consider bringing your pet to work. Why not lower your stress levels in the office as well as at home?

• Ask your friends to **share their special or funny pet stories**. They will warm your heart.

• If you want to see a touching and beautiful story, go to *www.youtube.com* and look up "Christian the Lion," a true story of a lion raised by two young men and then sent back to the wild.

*"The purity of a person's heart can be quickly measured by
how they regard animals."*
Anonymous

Instant Stress Reliever # 13 Go On Vacation
It Can Save Your Life!

"Vacation used to be a luxury, however, in today's world,
it has become a necessity."
Unknown

What is the number one killer of women in the world today? Heart disease. Did you know that if women aged 45-64 took two weeks of vacation a year, they would **cut the incidence of heart attacks in half!** [1] That's right, the simple act of going on vacation can save your life.

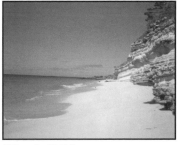

© Snowden McFall

Why is this such a difficult concept for Americans to grasp? Europeans have long known the value of "holiday." Most European countries give their employees 19 - 30+ vacation days yearly. The French typically receive about 38 vacation days a year and often take at least a month off at a time to unwind. It's expected and it's smart, for several reasons, from improved health and relationships to greater productivity.

But Americans tend to be workaholics. A Boston College study found that 26% of Americans **don't take any vacation at all** [2] and Reuters found that number had jumped to 43%. The 2013 Expedia study found most Americans don't take four of their paid vacation days. 59% of Americans feel vacation-deprived.[3] The Japanese are even worse. They have a name for death by overworking: karoshi. Over 150 cases of karoshi are reported annually and a lawsuit in late 2009 reported the death of a 41 year old female manager who had worked over 80 hours of overtime a month for the six months preceding her death.[4] Sadly, that is not unusual in Japan; 92% of the Japanese workforce do not take all of their vacation days.

Many of the groups I speak to say they are just too busy; they worry about what would happen to their work if they were gone. What you really should be worrying about is what will happen to you if you don't get some downtime. There is also evidence that you will be better at your job when you get some distance from it!

The Value of Vacations: You Make More Money and Your Productivity Goes Up!

According to Expedia, 34% of employed Americans say they return from vacation feeling better about their jobs and are **even more productive.** 53% say they come back feeling **rested and rejuvenated** after vacation. And 53% say they return home feeling reconnected with their family after a vacation. The Arizona Department of Health and Human Services found that women who took vacations were more satisfied with their marriages.[5] Lots of great reasons to take time away, aren't there?

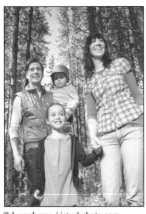

© bravobravo / istockphoto.com

Here are a few more. Dan Sullivan runs a Toronto company called Strategic Coach and requires his clients to take several vacations each year. In a survey of 3000 clients, Sullivan found that after 3 years, each client had doubled their annual free days and **doubled their income**! [6] Can you imagine what your life would be like if you doubled your income, especially in this economy?

Think about it. When you last returned from a good, restful vacation, didn't you feel more productive and effective at work? And consider your creative problem-solving. Did you come up with any new ideas or fresh solutions to business issues? Red Frog gives unlimited vacation days to their employees and no one ever abuses it. The company knows it increases productivity, performance. and creative thinking.

Almost every time, I have returned from vacations rested, relaxed and truly Fired Up! about my work. Sometimes my mind will quiet long enough for me to truly listen, and then I am amazed at what comes forward. I've come up with entire outlines for new books, innovative concepts for clients, designs for new artwork, just a variety of creativity rushing forth. For me, that rest and relaxation time is as essential as air and water. It renews my creative spirit and fills me with fresh, exciting concepts.

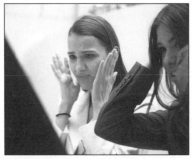

© webphotographer / istockphoto.com

Working On Vacation? Don't

One in four people plans to work while away; this is **not** a vacation. You have to let your mind rest and forget about work. **DO NOT** take your laptop or cellphone! 67% of Americans check email and voicemail on vacation, according to Expedia. That does NOT rest your mind. One international corporation I speak for learned that they couldn't get Internet service on certain cruises. All of sudden, there was a large increase in vacations on those cruises from that company! Seriously, it defeats the purpose of a vacation if you are in touch with the office the whole time. You have to let your mind and body truly unwind and enjoy. Plus your family will appreciate it if you leave work behind.

Vacations on a Budget: How to Take One in a Down Economy

There are many creative ways to take a vacation when money is tight. Here are a few:

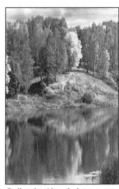

• Ask friends if you can **borrow their beach house or lake cabin**. Most people are very generous and would love to have you use their place. Just be sure to take excellent care of it, leave it sparkling clean, restocked and send them a nice thank you gift. Try to return the favor somehow, babysitting, etc.

© disapier / istockphoto.com

• **Consider bartering**- trading your services with a resort or someone who has a timeshare. One of my clients hired me to speak twice but could only afford my fee once. The second time, they paid me with a stay at a beautiful oceanfront resort. It gave me a much needed break and everything was paid for. We both won with the arrangement.

• Just **swap houses** with someone for a while. Again, take very good care of the home and leave it clean. It's a bit of an adventure, sleeping somewhere new and having a fresh environment. Obviously, there must be real trust there.

• **Plan a stay-cation**. That means staying at home at night but taking different trips during the day to places you normally never go. We had our nephew visiting and we took him to NASA at Cape Canaveral. It was exciting, fun, and something we had never done, even though we live only a few hours away.

Get creative. Find ways to have fun, whether it's playing new games at the beach, exploring local state parks, or visiting museums. Let go of the world of work for at least seven days. The benefits of vacation are enormous, for both you, your workplace, and your family. Don't shortchange any of them: take your vacations!

"By and large, mothers and housewives are the only workers who do not have regular time off. They are the great vacationless class."
Anne Morrow Lindbergh

Instant Stress Reliever # 14 Optimism
Think Positive, You Could Live Longer

*"Optimism is the one quality more associated with success
and happiness than any other."*
Brian Tracy

How is your day going? Are you feeling good, optimistic, excited about the future? Or are you tired, frustrated and overwhelmed? Does it seem like things are not getting any better? Believe it or not, your attitude makes a huge difference in your life, according to many brain researchers and experts like Dr. Daniel Amen. I love the story Michael J. Fox tells of a woman in Mozambique whose village flooded, and she gave birth in a tree. Whenever his children whine, he says *"A lady had a baby in a tree- whataddya got?"* That attitude is so typical of Michael, who has inspired so many in his battle with Parkinsons.[1a]

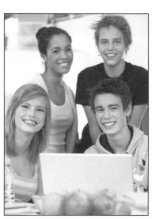

© Yuri Arcurs / istockphoto.com

What you focus on is what manifests in your life, so put your attention on what you want, not on what you don't want.

🕐 *When in debt, many people look at the growing pile of bills and their inability to pay them off and feel upset and demoralized. There have certainly been times in my life when I made this mistake. Instead, try this. Focus on the money you do have coming in and be grateful for the blessings in your life. And if you don't have a job, be thankful you have food, shelter and clothing. Thank your loved ones for being in your life, and thank your higher power for your health and home. When you put your energy into what you have and your appreciation for it, you create more of that. Focus instead on wealth in its many definitions. Recognize that you have great talents and blessings and use those to change direction.*

More Reasons to Think Positive

Optimists live seven years longer than pessimists, according to a study done at Yale University analyzing 600 people. Those who viewed aging from a positive perspective live on average 7.5 years longer than those who did not.

That means that just by having a more positive attitude, you can live nearly a decade longer.

Optimism has substantial health benefits. How's your breathing? Do you have asthma or frequent bronchitis? A study at Harvard found that optimists have significantly better lung function.[1] How is your attitude? Changing the way you feel about things may help you to breathe easier, literally.

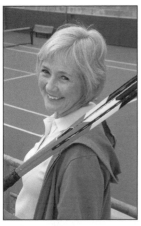

The National Institutes of Health studied 100,000 women and discovered that there is a strong correlation between optimism and a person's risk of death from cancer, heart disease, or early demise. Pessimistic women had a 23% higher risk of dying from a cancer-related condition.[2] You've heard that attitude is everything; when it comes to your health and longevity, it's the truth.

© jwblinn / istockphoto.com

Optimism in the Workplace

Given the economic pressures many areas of the world have encountered recently, how does optimism play out at work? No matter what the economy is doing, there are always certain people who thrive. Why do you think that is? It all has to do with attitude and perspective.

Dr. Martin Sullivan of the University of Pennsylvania spent 20 years interviewing 350,000 executives and learned something fascinating: **the top 10% performers think differently from others: they are all optimists!** That's a pretty amazing statistic. So if you want greater success, achievement, and effectiveness at work, become a more positive thinker.

Optimists take more risks and are more confident. Optimism is one of the core traits required in developing resilience, which is a critical factor in overcoming challenges and unexpected problems.[3] How about you? Can you bounce back easily from hard times?

How Pessimists Think and Why it Hurts Them

Pessimists and cynics tend to distrust others and be more suspicious of others and circumstances. They look for hidden agendas and hostile motives. They actually expect others to mistreat or betray them and that is exactly what happens. Sadly, this also backfires on them physically, as those who measure high on hostility scales are 25% more likely to develop heart disease. That's because they experience greater stress, which can cause a spike in an immune system protein called C3, which is linked to many diseases, including diabetes.[4]

> *"A pessimist sees the difficulty in every opportunity;*
> *an optimist sees the opportunity in every difficulty."*
> Winston Churchill

So What Do You Do If You're Pessimistic?

There's good news. **Optimism is only 25% inherited as a trait, so that means it is 75% learned.**[5]
That means if you tend to be a gloom and doom person, you can actually train yourself to have a more positive outlook. The University of MA found accident victims who were suddenly paralyzed were more optimistic than lottery winners.[6] Obviously, they had to train themselves to approach life from a new outlook and maintain an upbeat view of the future. So how do **you** begin to do that?

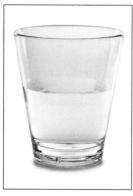

© skodonnell / istockphoto.com

One way is to **read inspiring stories** of people who have overcome shattering life experiences and continued to thrive. Here is a story of a friend of mine.

🕐 *All her life, Kim's mother verbally abused her and assaulted her self-esteem. No matter how loving Kim was, no matter how she excelled in school, Kim received bitter, negative comments from her mother. Even so, Kim stayed in touch with her family as an adult. In January 2008, Kim's mother was diagnosed with stage 4 cancer, and despite continued criticism, Kim took her mother to doctors' appointments and cared for her. Her father, a navy vet, was due to retire from the post office in a few years and was excited about a mortgage nearly paid off. News of his wife's cancer devastated him. Then he learned his wife had incurred $50,000 of new debt, which plunged him into a depression. One day in 2009, Kim went to pick up her mother for a doctor's appointment and could not get into the house. When the police finally broke in, they discovered a gruesome murder-suicide. Overwhelmed with grief and depression, her father had shot his wife and killed himself. And if that weren't shattering enough, they left a legacy of debt and bitterness. The $50,000 had become $100,000 and Kim found notebooks of nasty emails from her mother to others, consistently berating Kim. Clearly, Kim's mother hated her, wanted her to know it and Kim has no idea why. In spite of all of this, Kim is settling her mother's estate, staying positive, running her businesses and being the upbeat person she has always been. To meet her, you would never know what she has endured. Certainly, if anyone has cause to feel sorry for herself, Kim does. But she copes by spending time with her precious grown daughters, good friends, her two Yorkies, and a special man. Kim celebrates the best in life. Prayers and* *encouragement from other positive people keep her going. She has every reason to be bitter and cynical, but instead she chooses optimism instead and her life is better for it.* You can make that same choice. Every day, the way you face your life is a choice. Choose well!

How to Boost Your Optimism

• **Take care of yourself**, physically and emotionally. Optimists tend to exercise more, eat better, don't smoke and are more proactive about their health.

• **Spend time around positive people**; they will rub off on you. Stop associating with negative people, the whiners of the world. (Misery does love company.) Most every workplace has an *"Ain't it awful club™"* that hangs out in the cafeteria and moans about how bad things are. Avoid that group studiously. Instead, **ask others, "What's the good news?"** Focus on the positive and see how your life changes.

• When a difficult situation arises, **try examining it from a new perspective.** What good could come from this? What outdated, dysfunctional systems or conditions now need to improve? What are the possible benefits?

• **Look back at your own life** and think about periods you tend to label traumatic. How did you ultimately benefit from the experience? How did it help you? What did you learn from the hard times? Would you appreciate your life now without them?

• **Use humor**. Laughter helps you to feel differently about everything. If it will be funny later, why not let it be funny now?

• **Read biographies** of people who have overcome tragedy and heartbreak. Michael J. Fox's book *Always Looking Up: The Adventures of an Incurable Optimist* is a good one to start with. Watch winner movies, like *Dolphin Tale 1 and 2, Heaven is for Real, The Blind Side, Mr. Holland's Opus, Flashdance, Rudy, The Natural, The Secret of My Success, VisionQuest.* Listen to inspirational stories from speakers like W. Mitchell and Chad Hymas. Read *Success!* Magazine.

"Optimism is the faith that leads to achievement. Nothing can be done without hope and confidence."
Helen Keller

Instant Stress Reliever # 15 Volunteerism
Your Stress Dissolves When You Help Someone Else

"Service is the highest form of consciousness on the planet."
John Roger

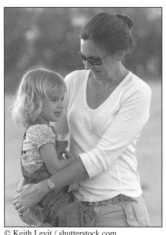

© Keith Levit / shutterstock.com

The Healing Power of Service

One of the last things you might think of doing when you are very stressed is to take the time to help someone else. But it can truly be the best thing you can do. I know this from my own personal experience.

Not too long ago, I was tired, frustrated and upset over a business issue. I was not sure how I was going to handle it. Heading home with my husband that night, we turned down our street. He said, "There's a girl sitting on the corner crying." We immediately stopped the car and I got out to talk to her. Turns out, she was working for one of those magazine sales companies where they drop off youths and pick them up at the end of the day. She had no phone and no money; her ride was two hours late. So we called her manager and he said a ride was on its way. She waited in the car with us, shared her tragic life story, and when no ride arrived after 45 minutes, we turned around and drove her the half hour distance to her motel. When we arrived, I spoke to the manager about taking better care of this young woman (she was 20,) gave her some money and hugged her goodbye with some encouraging words. As we drove home again, all thoughts about my problems had completely vanished. My concerns were for her and how I could help others like her in the future. I realized my problems were far less pressing. There are those who are struggling to get by every day on the streets. It gave me a whole new appreciation of how fortunate I am.

That's the value of volunteerism. It gives you perspective, awareness of how blessed your life really is, and it gets you out of the worry and anxiety of stress.

The Benefits of Volunteerism

There are several benefits of community service.
Volunteering:
• promotes connection and sharing
• decreases stress and depression
• improves interpersonal skills
• enhances communication skills
• increases gratitude and empathy
• improves understanding of community issues[1]
• strengthens your ability to cope
• makes you feel good about yourself and
  your gifts and talents
• increases how long you live [2]
• provides a sense of fulfillment and purpose
• strengthens the community

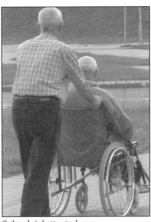
© thumb / shutterstock.com

Cornell University conducted a study on the impact of environmental volunteerism on seniors, and discovered that those who volunteer outside became more physically active and benefitted from the added stress reduction of being in nature. They had more energy, a greater ability to cope, and stronger emotional well-being. Younger nature volunteers had increased concentration, reduced aggression, decreased stress and improved self-esteem.[3]

Volunteerism in the US

62.6 million people, or 25.4% of the US population, volunteered for an organization at least once between Sept. 2012 and Sept. 2013. 27.2% of all employed people volunteered and 24.1% of the unemployed volunteered.[4]

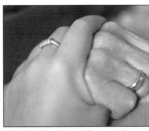
© Natalia Bratslavsky / Shutterstock

There are infinite ways to volunteer:
• mentor a child
• help a neighbor repair their home
• organize a fundraiser for the arts
• work at a soup kitchen
• help at a homeless shelter
• participate in a "clean up your park" project
• volunteer at an animal shelter
• read to seniors at a senior center or hospital
• collect diapers for newborn centers
• help out at elementary schools
• collect books for literacy programs and then read for them

- run a food drive for local food banks
- teach some craft or art skill to children or seniors
- give clothes and supplies to a local battered women's shelter
- help out at an after-school day care center
- count birds for a local wildlife sanctuary

One of my favorite volunteering experiences came from my work with Professional Women's Council. We organized a group to participate in "Adopt a Room," a program of Community Connections in Jacksonville, FL, which provides housing to women and children who have been homeless. Residents must have a job to stay at the facility. These folks arrive with nothing and are given a bed and a bureau. We provide the sheets, blankets and all decor for these rooms, from cosmetic items like shampoo, to curtains, bedspreads, mirrors, pillows, art, bathrobes, slippers

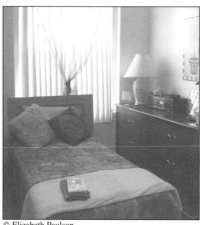
© Elizabeth Paulson

and chachkas, all of which they get to keep when they leave. My favorite story came a few days after we had been there to decorate some rooms. A young woman who graduated out of the foster care system moved in and was given the keys to her room. She promptly returned to the front desk and said, "This can't be my room - someone else is living there. The front desk attendant accompanied her upstairs and looked around and said,"Honey, this is your room. Some people were here this weekend and decorated it for you." At which point, she burst into tears and said she had never had anyone do anything like that for her. She loved it and was so happy. Of course, when we all heard the story, there were more tears of joy and a deep feeling of gratitude to have been able to do something like that for her.

That's the power of volunteering. It has an incredible impact on your health, longevity and stress levels. For me, it is absolutely one of the best instant stress relievers around, and you can do it at any time, any place, anywhere.

*"Too often we underestimate the power of a touch, a smile, a kind word,
a listening ear, an honest compliment, or the smallest act of caring,
all of which have the potential to turn a life around."*
Leo Buscaglia

10 Ways to Stay Fired Up!
and Prevent Burnout

1. **Do something you love every day**. Schedule in what brings you joy.

2. **Set a timer** throughout your work day. At least once an hour, get up, drink water, stretch your shoulders, neck and wrists, and talk to someone.

3. **Ask for help**, with projects at work and at home. Teams work together.

4. **Create a "Feel-Good" Folder** on your desktop or as a paper folder of cartoons, postcards, cards from loved ones, vacation spots, etc. to cheer you on tough days.

5. **Spend time in nature**, regularly. Walk in the woods, on a beach, by a lake, near a tree.

6. **Avoid negative people,** bad news, and pessimists.

7. **Connect with something larger than yourself every day**. It could be the purity of a baby's smile, God, or whatever works for you.

8. **Celebrate victories large and small**, with others!

9. **Be kind to yourself when you make a mistake**. Forgive yourself and let it go. Recall your successful moments and realize you will have more.

10. **Keep learning new things**, trying new skillsets and stretching out of your comfort zone. Share what you learn.

About the Author

Snowden McFall is an inspirational and dynamic speaker, trainer and author. Founder and president of Brightwork Advertising and Training, Inc., a full service ad agency opened in 1983, and Fired Up! a professional speaking business since 1996, Snowden's trademark qualities are her enthusiasm, authenticity and her ability to get people "*Fired Up!*" Speaking for companies like Fidelity National Financial, YMCA, Pfizer, Vistakon, First Citizens Bank, Blue Cross Blue Shield, Allstate, and Helms Briscoe, Snowden is a business expert who speaks on motivation, stress management, teambuilding, volunteerism and productivity. She has authored and co-authored 5 books, including *Fired Up!*, which has sold over 65,000 copies worldwide.

Snowden is a passionate community trustee. She was named the "**National Women in Business Advocate of the Year" by the Small Business Administration for her nonprofit work helping female entrepreneurs.** As a result, Snowden was honored at a Rose Garden Ceremony at the White House and a Congressional luncheon. A finalist for *Inc.* Magazine's "New England Entrepreneur of the Year," Snowden is an active member of the Jacksonville, FL Regional Chamber of Commerce. She has served on the Women's Business Center Athena Powerlink panels and as a mentor for Marketing Matters. A board member of Professional Women's Council, she chairs the Community Involvement Committee. A former board member of Women Business Owners, she is a member of the National Speakers Association and Meeting Professionals International. A member of the Jacksonville Womens Network, Snowden was voted Small Business Leader of the Year by the Professional Women's Council. A 2010 Leadership Jacksonville graduate, Snowden received President Obama's Presidential Volunteer Service Award for her community service. In 2014, the *Jacksonville Business Journal* chose her as a Woman of Influence in the community.

Snowden has appeared on 320 radio shows, **CNN Financial News, Bloomberg Television,** and The Home Shopping Network. Quoted in *Investors Business Daily*, *Foxnews.com* and *Success* Magazine as an expert on burnout, Snowden has a blog at www.firedupnow.com/blog, and regularly comments on Twitter, Linkedin and Facebook. Snowden is married and loves to go to the beach, travel, write, dance and entertain.

Other Products and Services

Snowden McFall has authored and co-authored 4 other books:
Fired Up! How to Succeed by Making Your Dreams Come True
(a private label version of that book)
Wholehearted Success
Exceptional Accomplishment

Audios as CDs or MP3s include:
Fire Up! Your Presentation Skills™
Stress and Change: Moving From Fear and Frustration to Fired Up!™
Find Your Happiness & Dramatically Improve Your Business Success™
Package
The Fired Up! Woman's Guide to Success™ Audio Series including audios on self-esteem, stress, marketing, and effective networking
The Fired Up! Make Your Dreams Come True Home Study™ course
Her complete line of books, audios, white papers, webinars, etc. can be found at www.firedupnow.com

Keynotes, Corporate Trainings and Custom Programs:

Stress Express! 15 Instant Stress Relievers ™
Get Fired Up! for Success™
Reignite the Fire and Prevent Burnout™ - Manage Stress & Thrive
Fan the Flames - Fire Up Your Team & Spark Productivity™
Fire Up! Your Business for Success™
Rekindle the Fire Within- Igniting Greatness in Women™
Rekindle the Core - Fire Up Your Employees for Success™

Snowden also does consulting, transition coaching and custom program design for clients. Learn more at www.firedupnow.com or call 1-888-FIREKBKS

Follow Snowden in Social Media:
http://twitter.com/snowdenmcfall
http://www.facebook.com/snowdenmcfall
http://www.linkedin.com/in/snowdenmcfall
http://www.youtube.com/snowdenmcfall

Footnotes

Introduction

1a. Aetna.com, "The Facts About Rising Health Care Costs"
http://www.aetna.com/health-reform-connection/aetnas-vision/facts-about-costs.html

1. Study by Stay Well Health Management published in April 2009 in the US cities:
http://www.twincities.com/ci_12169155?source=most_emailed

2. "Stress in US Rises, Causes Health Problems," The Scoop, *The Meeting Professional*, March 2008, p.44

3. Jourdain, Kathy and Tangri , Ravi, "The Corporate Costs of Stress," Crysalis, Sept. 2001. Vol 2. No. 2, *www.cocreatingfutures.com*

4. Anschuetz, Barbara L. Dr, "The High Cost of Caring- Coping with Workplace Stress," http://www.epilepsyontario.org/client/EO/EOWeb.nsf/web/The+High+Cost+of+Caring+-+Workplace+Stress

5. "Stress Feeds Cancer," *WRCB TV Channel 3*, July 8, 2009
http://www.wrcbtv.com/Global/story.asp?S=10661285

6. Caminiti, Susan, "Work-Life," *Fortune Magazine,* Sept. 19, 2005, p.S8

7. Forster, Julie, "Study shows benefits of keeping workers health," *TwinCities.com*, April 17, 2009 study by Stay Well Health Management

8. *American Journal of Preventive Medicine,* Dec 2005

9. Merritt, Richard, "Stress Management Significantly Reduces Long-term Costs of Coronary Artery Disease," American Psychological Association

10. Young, Joyce, "IBM's Well-Being Director," *Benefit News*, March 2006

11 Kennedy, John M,. "How Reducing Stress in the Workplace Saves Dollars and Lives," Feb 9, 2010, *Sales and Marketing.com*

12 Forbes Staff, "Most Effective Stress Relievers, *Forbes.com,* November. 9, 2009

13. Ozminkowski RJ, Dunn RL, Goetzel RZ, Cantor RI, Murnane J, Harrison M. A "Return on Investment Evaluation of the Citibank, N.A., Health Management Program." *American Journal Health Promotion,* Sep/Oct 1999: 5(I14).

Chapter 1 Relax Your Jaw

1. 3. & 5. Yardegaran, Jessica, "Grinding Your Teeth? It's Stress, "*The Mercury News.com*, Nov. 16, 2009 (San Jose, CA Mercury News)

2. "Grinding Away Stress with Your Teeth?" The Early Show, *CBS News*, Oct. 9, 2009

4. Weinstein, Lee, "Saving Your Teeth and Protecting Your Wallet," 2009 Ebook
http://stopgrinding.com/

6. Melinda Beck, "When Stress Sets Your Teeth on Edge," for *Associated Press*, 12/1/08 *The Pottstown Mercury,* PA

Chapter 2 Sleep

1. *Neurobiology of Aging* February 18, 2014 [Epub ahead of print]
http://articles.mercola.com/sites/articles/archive/2014/09/18/poor-sleep-causes-brain-damage.aspx?e_cid=20140918Z1_DNL_art_1&utm_source=dnl&utm_medium=email&utm_content=art1&utm_campaign=20140918Z1&et_cid=DM55895&et_rid=663357121

2. Sharma, Sanchita, "Sleep on this at your own risk," *Hindustan Times*, June 20, 2009,
http://www.hindustantimes.com/News-Feed/newdelhi/Sleep-on-this-at-your-own-risk/Article1-421255.aspx

3. Edwards, Laurie "Your sleep and your health," *Glamour.com*, June 2008, p.96

4.and 7. Fisher, Anne, Overfelt, Maggie and Sraswat, Shuchi, "Make sleep work for you," *Fortune Small Business*, Sept. 2008, p.86-90
http://money.cnn.com/2008/08/19/smallbusiness/make_sleep_work_for_you.fsb/index.htm

5. & 14. Schwab, Dave, "Study: Naps improves brain power," *La Jolla Light*, CA, April 1, 2009

6. *PR Web*, "Top 5 Ways to Getting Better Quality Sleep, May 30, 2012

7. Thakur, Duke University Medical Center 2004 and "Snooze Flash," Health News, *Ladies Home Journal*, May, 2009, p.144 University of Chicago Medical Center Study

8. Knight, Jobee, "Studies Find Stress Causes Chronic Insomnia, Depletes Calcium," November 22, 2009, http://sleepapneadisorder.info/?p=1331

9. Wilkie, Ross, *Reuters*, February 19, 2014

10. Kelly, Trista, "You lose if you don't snooze: lost sleep can't be recovered," *Business Week*, Jan. 13, 2010, http://www.businessweek.com/news/2010-01-13/you-lose-if-you-don-t-snooze-lost-sleep-can-t-be-recovered.html

11. "Sleep Deprivation Rise at Work, *BBC News*, June 21, 2005
http://news.bbc.co.uk/2/hi/uk_news/wales/4114876.stm

12. and 14. Hyatt, Michael, "5 Reasons Why You Should Take a Nap Every Day," blogpost 2012 http://michaelhyatt.com/why-you-should-take-a-nap-every-day.html#comment-479354249

13. Rich-Kern, Sheryl, "Napping At Work Becoming Part of Corporate Culture?" *New Hampshire Public Radio,* August 6, 2008 http://www.nhpr.org/node/16986

15. HealthyandNaturalWorld,.com, "23 Dangers of Sleep Deprivation," Feb.24, 2014
http://www.healthyandnaturalworld.com/dangers-of-sleep-deprivation/

16. Fisher, Anne, "In praise of the power nap," *Fortune Small Business*, August 25, 2008
http://money.cnn.com/2008/08/19/smallbusiness/power_nap.fsb/index.htm

17. Mercola, Dr.,"Lack of Sleep May Lead to Brain Shrinkage,"*Mercola.com,* Sept. 20, 2014
http://articles.mercola.com/sites/articles/archive/2014/09/18/poor-sleep-causes-brain-damage.aspx?e_cid=20140918Z1_DNL_art_1&utm_source=dnl&utm_medium=email&utm_content=art1&utm_campaign=20140918Z1&et_cid=DM55895&et_rid=663357121

Chapter 3 Eat the Right Food

1. "Obesity and Overweight," World Health Organization website
http://www.who.int/dietphysicalactivity/publications/facts/obesity/en/

2. Warner, Jennifer, "Stress Unlocks Fat Cells, Ups Obesity: Study Shows Molecule Released During Stress May Unlock Body's Fat Cells," *WebMD Health News*, July 2, 2007

3. "Pet Obesity Facts and Risks," Association for Pet Obesity Prevention, July 20, 2009
http://www.petobesityprevention.com/facts.htm

4. Gorrell, Carin "Is Stress Making You Fat?" *Redbook* reprinted in *San Francisco Chronicle,* July 16, 2009, p.83, http://tinyurl.com/l7

5. "Belly Off! 2008: Success Stories, The Best At-Home Health Test," *Men's Health,* December 2008 http://tinyurl.com/kp4dtu

6. "Eat your way happy and healthy," *Woman's World*, May 5, 2008, p.12 http://www.harvard-science.harvard.edu/medicine-health/articles/food-ingredients-may-be-effective-antidepressants

7. "Tuna boosts your optimism," *Woman's World*, May 5, 2008, p.12 According to Harvard researcher James Hudson, MD

8. "Wonderfoods that help keep the doctor away," *Weather.com* (LifeWire) Feb. 19. 2008

9. "Tired All Summer," *First* Magazine, August 20, 2007

10. Honey: The index of medical and scientific journals at the National Medical Library in Bethesda, Md.

11. "Smart Ideas to Make Life Happier: Eat a Worry-Busting Breakfast," *Womens World*, May 5, 2008, p.3

12. "Stress Reduction and Chi: Ultimate Green Tea Extract," Tea Psychopharmacology Study, 2007, *Ultimate Green Tea Blog,* Dec. 10, 2008

13. "The Healing Power of Tea," *Ladies Home Journal,* Feb. 2009, p.38

14. Alleyne, Richard, " A cup of tea really can help reduce stress at times of crisis," *Telegraph.co.uk,* August 13, 2009

15. Lamb, Ed, "Chocolate may prevent deadly strokes," *Norfolk Health Care Examiner,* February 13, 2010 http://www.examiner.com/x-15966-Norfolk-Health-Care-Examiner~y2010m2d13-Chocolate-may-prevent-deadly-strokes

16. King, Margie, "Dark Chocolate Relieves Stress," *www.greenmedinfo.com,* Sept. 26, 2012 http://www.greenmedinfo.com/blog/dark-chocolate-relieves-stress-and-lowers-blood-pressure

Chapter 4 Aromatherapy

1. Worwood, Valerie Ann, *The Fragrant Mind*, Bantam Books, London, 1997

2. "Smart You Solutions: Ensure Everyone Gets Along," *First for Women*, May 3, 2010, p.4

3. "Happiness Scents." *Woman's World*, August 4, 2008, p.20

4. "Smart Ideas to Kiss Your Worries Goodbye," *Woman's World*, Oct.15, 2012, p.3

5. "Cure the Car-Trip Crankies: Banish a Bad Mood," *First*, June 30, 2008, p.100

6. "Decorate with These for More Holiday Happiness," *Woman's World,* Dec. 8, 2008, p.17

7. Hall, Susan. "The other reasons to love flowers" *Health.com,* April 2008
Study by Havilland-Jones, study at Harvard Medical School and study at Texas A&M.
http://www.aromatherapygoddess.com/aromatherapyfacts.html
http://www.aromatherapy-stress-relief.com/stressatwork.html

Chapter 5 Water

1. and 4. "11 Reasons Dehydration is Making You Sick and Fat, *TheMindUnleashed.com,* Sept.11, 2014 http://themindunleashed.org/2014/09/11-reasons-dehydration-making-sick-fat.html

2. Emoto, Masaru, "Introduction," *The Hidden Messages in Water*, Beyond Words Publishing, 2004, p.xv

3. Beuermann-King, Beverly, "Water : A Necessity in Maintaining Mental Health," July 20, 2009, *www.WorkSmartLiveSmart.com*

5. Prevention.com, "Just Add Water," March 2014

6. Seah, David, "The Healing Power of Water," *www.davidseah.com* http://davidseah.com/blog/the-healing-power-of-water/

7 and 9. Cuffey, Abigail and Kirkwood, Judy, "H2ohhh," *Ladies Home Journal,* August 2008, p.26-27

8. Khoto, William, "The Healing Power of a Simple Bath," *Ezinearticles.com* http://ezinearticles.com/?The-Healing-Power-of-a-Simple-Bath&id=1278449

10. Website of Masaru Emoto: http://www.masaru emoto.net/english/e_ome_annai.html

11. Dr. Mercola, "Can Water Go Bad? Sept. 22, 2014, *www.mercola.com*
http://articles.mercola.com/sites/articles/archive/2014/09/22/can-water-go-bad.aspx?e_cid=20140922Z1_DNL_art_1&utm_source=dnl&utm_medium=email&utm_content=art1&utm_ca mpaign=20140922Z1&et_cid=DM56405&et_rid=667289584

Chapter 6 Yoga and Exercise

1. and 3. Lind, Dr. Peter, "Yoga and Stress." *www.therapeuticreiki.com*
http://therapeuticreiki.com/blog/yoga-and-stress/

2. Avery, Sarah, "Studies show yoga can treat illness," *McClatchy Newspapers,* Nov. 28, 2008

4. "Reach for It, " *Prevention Magazine*, p.14, November 2013

5. Lisica, Flora, "Yoga helps war veterans with PTSD," *The Conversation*, Sept. 15. 2014

6. Hoffman, Matthew, MD, "The Health Benefits of Yoga." *WebMD.com*, August 12, 2008
http://www.webmd.com/balance/the-health-benefits-of-yoga and "Yoga," A *PubMEd*, Duke University, November 11, 2008

7. *"Live Longer," Women's World,* May 5, 2008, p. 15

8. Orme-Johnson, *Psychosomatic Medicine* 49 (1987) Meditators showed hospitalization rates 87% less than non-meditators for heart disease, 55% less for benign and malignant tumors, 30% less for infectious diseases, and 50% less for out-patient doctor visits.

9. Jacobs, Harvard Medical, "Say Goodnight To Insomnia," *Owl Books* (1999)

10. Harrison, *Clinical Child Psychology and Psychiatry 9* (4) (October, 2004)
48 children in a 6-week meditation program with an average 35% improvement in ADHD symptoms. Of 31 children taking medication, 11 were able to reduce it.

11. 1998 study, *Journal of American Medical Association,* showed that meditation paired with low-fat, whole foods, vegetarian diet and aerobic exercise, lowers the risk of heart attacks.

Chapter 7 Creative Expression

1a. Health: "Picture Yourself Resilient," *Prevention*, October, 2014, p.17

1. Health and Body Book,"How to Live to 100, *Glamour,* June 2008, p.95

2. Siedliecki, Sandra L., PhD RN CNS, and Good, Marion. PhD RN, "Effect of music on power, pain, depression and disability," *Journal of Advanced Nursing* Volume 54 Issue 5, pgs.553 - 562 Published Online: 22 May 2006 © 2010 Blackwell Publishing

3.&4. "Making music improves your health: FACT!" Dec. 3, 2008
http://musicianstools.wordpress.com,

5. Hall, Susan, "The Best Stay-Young Secret Yet," Healthy Life, *Health.com* May 2008, p.89

Chapter 8 Anger

1a.Wolt, Hannah, "Surprising News About Anger," *Prevention,* June 2013, p.22

1. and 3. "Controlling Anger -- Before It Controls You" http://www.apa.org/topics/controlanger.html
American Psychological Association article

2. Rosenberg, Marshall, Ph.D., *Non-Violent Communication*, http://www.cnvc.org

4a. "Enjoy Two More Years by Letting Off Steam," *Woman's World*, March 18, 2013, p.13

4. Vermond, Kira, " A little anger is not always a bad thing," *Money Talks*, March 23, 2009
discussing Harvard Study of Adult Development
http://www.cbc.ca/money/moneytalks/2009/03/kira_vermond_a_little_anger_is.html

5. "Nails in the Fence," Author Unknown
http://www.inspirationpeak.com/cgi-bin/stories.cgi?record=50 author unknown

6. Mills, Harry, Ph.D, "Physiology of Anger," *MentalHelp.net*, June 25, 20005
http://www.mentalhelp.net/poc/view_doc.php?type=doc&id=5805&cn=116

7. Boerma, Christina, "The Physiology of Anger," Healthmad, *Presstv.com, August 12, 2007*
http://www.healthmad.com/Mental-Health/Physiology-of-Anger.38920 H

8. Marcus, Mary Brophy, " Health Update: How Anger Makes You Sick," *Self.com,* May 2008, p.187

9. "Emotional Stress Linked to Elderly Falls," study in *BMC Geriatrics,* March 1, 2009

10. If you are experiencing domestic violence, get help. National Domestic Violence Hotline (www.ndvh.org) call the National Domestic Violence Hotline 1-800-799-SAFE(7233)

11. Fennessy, Donna, " I'm Sorry - How to Deal with Angry People," *Self,* April 2001, p.127

Chapter 9 Laughter

1. "Mirthful laughter," *APS.org* Study by Dr. Lee Berk, DRPH, MPH at the 122nd Annual Meeting of the American Physiological Society

2. http://www.associatedcontent.com/article/624637/laughterthe_health_benefits.html?cat=5

2a. Mayo Clinic Staff, "Stress Management," www.mayoclinic.org,
http://www.mayoclinic.org/healthy-living/stress-management/in-depth/stress-relief/art-20044456?p=1

3. www.webmd.com/guide/give-your-body-boost-with-laughter

4. Laughter research and laughter clubs http://risatel.blogspot.com/ and http://www.laughteryoga.org/

5. Loma Linda School of Public Health
http://humanresources.about.com/od/stressandtimemanagement/a/laughter.htm, http://www.bellaonline.com/articles/art29733.asp

6. Tracz, Pam "Laughter Programs," http://www.laughingisgoodforyou.com/programs.htm

7. Granirer, David, "Laughing Your Way to Organizational Health: A Lighter Approach to Workplace Wellness," for *About.com*

Chapter 10 Friendship

1a. El Nasser, Haya, and Overberg, Paul, "More people choose to go solo." *USA Today.com,* Oct. 10, 2012

1. & 2 Kleinfield, Judith, "The effects of loneliness are serious, studies show," *Fairbanks Daily News Mirror,* April 5, 2009

3. Harms, William, "Isolation and stress identified as contributing to breast cancer risk,"
www.eurekalert.org http://www.eurekalert.org/pub_releases/2009-12/uoc-ias120309.php

4. and 9. Taylor, S. E.; Klein, L.C.; Lewis, B. P.; Gruenewald, T. L.; Gurung, R. A. R.; & Updegraff, J. A. "Female Responses to Stress: Tend and Befriend, Not Fight or Flight", *Psychological Review* (2000), 107(3), p.41-429.

5. Farquhar, Amelia, "Boost your brainpower by calling a friend," *Women's World*, Dec. 8, 2008

6. "Make a Date with a Friend," *Good Housekeeping*, Jan. 2013, p. 101

7. McCafferty, Megan, "Easy Ways to Add Years to Your Life" and "Where Did All My Friends Go?" *Ladies Home Journal*, Feb., 2009, p. 140 and *Health.com*, April 2008

8. "You+Friends= Better Health," *Prevention Magazine*, December 2013, p. 18

10. Weiner, Staci, "The how of happiness," *Good Housekeeping*, March 27, 2009
http://www.seattlepi.com/health/403362_goodhouse272799.html?source=mypi

11. Higson-Hughes, Kristin, "How far would you go for a friend?" *Womans World,* December 8, 2008, p.54

12. Johnson, Carolyn, "Happiness has its own network," *Boston.com*, December 4, 2008

13. Kotz, Deborah, "Love and Romance: Get the Health Benefits Even if You're Single", *US News & World Report*, February 13, 2009, Univ. of Virginia study

Chapter 11 Completion

1. White, Martha, " 5 Scientifically Proven Ways to Reduce Stress at Work," *Time.com*
http://business.time.com/2014/01/22/5-scientifically-proven-ways-to-reduce-stress-at-work

2. Fritz, Robert, *The Path of Least Resistance*, Stillpoint Publishing, October 1986

3. The concept of broken agreements is explored fully in Insight® Seminars Training.

Chapter 12 Pets

1. Brown, Geoff, 'Tails of Love," *AARP* Magazine, Nov./Dec., 2009

2. Cotthart, Melissa "Fluffy to the Rescue," *AARP* Magazine Sept./Oct. 2008

3. "People May Draw More Support from Furry Friends than Spouses, Human Allies," *Health Behavior News Service*, Sept. 25, 2002, www.newswise.com/articles/view/31716/

4. & 5. Scott, Elizabeth, "How Owning a Dog or Cat Can Reduce Stress," *About.com Guide*, Sept.6, 2009 http://stress.about.com/od/lowstresslifestyle/a/petsandstress.htm

Chapter 13 Vacations

1. and 2. and 6. Brown, Sarah, "Clean Break," *Vogue,* June 2003

3. "2013 International Vacation Deprivation ™ Survey," *Expedia.com*
http://viewfinder.expedia.com/features/2013-vacation-deprivation-study

4. "McDonald's Worker Dies of Overwork," *Google News,* Oct. 27, 2009 ©2010 AFP
http://www.google.com/hostednews/afp/article/ALeqM5gwgGnPxcowg7_
uyZJCFFGXnT1N6w

5. Scott, Elizabeth, M.S, "The Importance of Vacations, for Stress Relief, Productivity and Health; Vacations Are Important For More Than Just Fun," *About.com Guide,* May 23, 2009
http://stress.about.com/od/workplacestress/a/vacations.htm

Chapter 14 Optimism

1a. Ellis, Rosemary, "No Complaints, No Excuses," *Good Housekeeping*, Oct. 2013, pp.39-44

1. and 3. Naish, John, " How to Think Yourself Successful," *TimesOnLine,* Jan. 3, 2009
Annual Review of Clinical Psychology Study by Dr. Becca Levy at Yale University of 660 volunteers. Harvard Medical Study of 670 men by Dr. Rosalind Wright

2. Cox, Lauren, "Pollyanna Will Outlive Everyone," *ABC News*, March 6, 2009,
http://abcnews.go.com/print?id=7017131

4. Vance, Allie "Seven Thoughts that are Bad for You," *Zikkir,* Sept. 13, 2009
http://zikkir.com/index/32268?wscr=1440x900

5. "Optimism" *Redbookmag.com*, May 2006, p.148

6. "The Secrets of Resilient Women," *Woman's Day.com,* April 1, 2008, p.74, Carolyn Kaufman, clinical psychologist at Columbus State Community College in Ohio

Chapter 15 Volunteerism

1. "National Survey of Giving, Volunteering and Participating: The Benefits of Volunteering," Canadian Centre for Philanthropy research Program, 2000 http://www.nationalservice.gov/about/volunteering/benefits.asp

2. "The Health Benefits of Volunteering," Corporation for National & Community Service, April 19, 2006 http://www.worldvolunteerweb.org/fileadmin/docdb/ pdf/2007/07_0506_USAbenefits_health.pdf

3. Bushway, Lori, et al. "Environmental Volunteerism as a Form of Civic Engagement for Older Adults: Benefits, Motivations and Barriers," Cornell University, www.citra.org/wordpress/wp-content/uploads/?ce.doc *www.cornell.edu*

4. "Volunteering in the United States, 2013," Bureau of Labor Statistics, Feb. 25, 2014 http://www.bls.gov/news.release/volun.nr0.html

For more information about Snowden McFall and her other books, audios, products, keynote speeches, corporate trainings and webinars, go to www.firedupnow.com Call 1-888-347-3257 or 904-940-7355.